# The Ultimate Anti-Inflammatory Cookbook

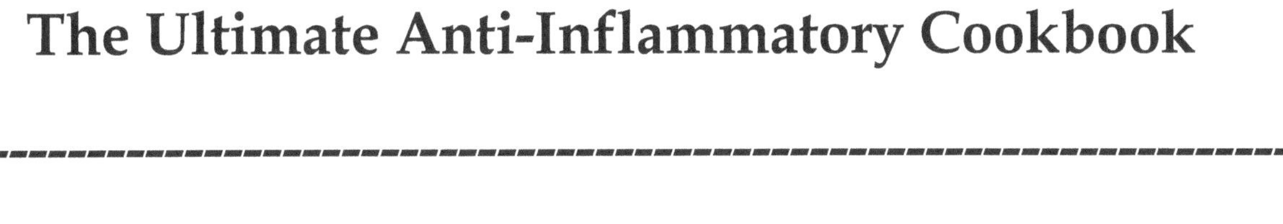

## Delicious Recipes to Reduce Inflammation and Improve Your Health

# Table of Contents

# Introduction

In today's fast-paced world, where worry, smog, and bad eating habits are common, chronic inflammation has become a common health problem. Inflammation is the body's normal response to damage and infection, but if it lasts for a long time, it can cause inflammatory diseases, heart disease, and gout, among other health problems.

The good news is that by consciously choosing the foods you consume, you may have control over your health and well-being. This cookbook serves as your how-to manual for preparing delectable, filling meals that not only fulfill your hunger but also aid your body's battle against inflammation.

You'll find a selection of delectable recipes on the pages that follow, each of which was thoughtfully created to incorporate foods with anti-inflammatory effects. These recipes are designed to make you feel your best and enjoy life to the fullest. They range from colorful salads to filling main dishes and guilt-free sweets.

This Cookbook contains something for everyone, whether you're unfamiliar with the idea of an anti-inflammatory diet or you're currently on it and seeking new inspiration. Here, we'll look at the science of inflammation, introduce you to several essential anti-inflammatory foods, and give you some useful advice on how to include them in your regular diet.

The food you place on your plate is the first step on your path to greater health. Discover the delicious tastes and health advantages of an anti-inflammatory diet with the help of this cookbook. Take up a new diet, discover how these dishes may change your life, and start your journey to a healthier, more energetic you. One tasty nibble at a time and your body will appreciate you for it.

Discover a healthier you with this Anti-Inflammatory Cookbook for Beginners! Start your journey towards wellness today—explore nourishing recipes, expert tips, and transformative meal plans to soothe inflammation. Embrace vibrant health with every delicious dish. Ready to embark on this flavorful healing adventure?

# Chapter 1: The Basics of Anti-Inflammatory Eating

## 1.1 Understanding Inflammation and its Impact on Health

An integral and important component of our body's protection mechanism is inflammation. It describes how our body reacts to wounds, infections, and outside invaders like viruses and bacteria. Chronic inflammation may be harmful to human health, but acute inflammation is an important and natural reaction that aids in healing and defense against possible dangers. In this post, we'll examine the many manifestations of inflammation, its root causes, and the wide-ranging effects they have on our general health and well-being.

### The two-pronged nature of inflammation

The coin of inflammation has two sides. On the one hand, acute inflammation is a rapid and under-control immunological response to a variety of stimuli. The body's approach of alerting you that something is wrong often appears as redness, heat, swelling, and discomfort. For instance, the damaged region gets inflamed when you acquire a cut or a splinter as white blood cells rush to the area to ward against infection and start the healing process.

On the other hand, chronic inflammation causes harm to our systems since it is a protracted and less localized reaction. Chronically, high levels of pro-inflammatory markers characterize it. It may be brought on by a variety of things, such as a poor diet, inactivity, ongoing stress, and exposure to pollutants in the environment.

### The root causes of persistent inflammation

1. Diet: What we consume greatly influences inflammation. Inflammation may be fueled by a diet heavy in processed foods, sweets, bad fats, and deficient in critical nutrients. On the other hand, an anti-inflammatory diet has a lot of whole foods, vitamins, and omega-3 fatty acids.

2. Insufficient exercise Adopting a sedentary lifestyle increases inflammation. It has been shown that regular exercise lowers inflammation by enhancing circulation and encouraging the production of anti-inflammatory chemicals.

Three. Chronic stress may make inflammation worse. Hormones that might induce inflammation when generated in excess are released as a result of stress. Maintaining low inflammation levels requires managing stress via relaxation methods, mindfulness, and social support.

4. Environmental pollutants Chronic inflammation may be brought on by pollution, heavy metals, and certain substances. The risk may be reduced by reducing exposure to certain poisons, such as by using air purification systems and avoiding particular compounds.

Five. Obesity: Fat tissue is metabolically active and creates pro-inflammatory chemicals, particularly around the belly. Chronic inflammation and obesity are closely related, and chronic inflammation has been linked to a number of diseases.

**The Effects of Long-Term Inflammation**

Several health issues are linked to chronic inflammation, including:

1. Heart illness: Atherosclerosis and blood vessel damage brought on by inflammation may raise the risk of heart attacks and strokes.

2. Cancer: Some malignancies are thought to begin and advance as a result of chronic inflammation.

3. Autoimmune Conditions Autoimmune diseases like Lupus and rheumatoid arthritis happen when the body's immune system attacks its tissues because of swelling.

4. Neurological Conditions: According to research, neurological illnesses like Alzheimer's and Parkinson's are linked to persistent inflammation.

5. **Problems with digestion:** Irritable Bowel Syndrome (IBS) and Crohn's disease may be made worse by stomach inflammation that lasts for a long time.

6. Diabetes: The body's reaction to insulin may be hampered by inflammation, which can result in insulin resistance and diabetes.

7. **Aging:** According to some studies, persistent inflammation speeds up aging on both the inside and the outside, causing problems including wrinkles and premature aging.

**Measurement and Control of Inflammation**

Monitoring inflammation levels is essential for optimal management. There are several tests that can measure CRP, ESR, and other things cytokines are a few typical assays. These tests may aid in determining if and how much inflammation there is inside the body.

*Changing one's lifestyle is usually necessary to manage inflammation:*

1. **Diet:** Eat a diet low in inflammatory foods, such as those found in fish, olive oil, and nuts, and high in A lot of fruits, veggies, and whole foods, lean protein, and good fats. Lessen your sugar, trans fats, and processed meals.

2. Exercise: Exercise on a regular basis to promote general health and minimize inflammation.

3. Stress Management: To successfully manage stress, try relaxation methods like yoga, deep breathing exercises, or meditation.

4. **Sleep:** Give sleep a priority since a lack of sleep can cause inflammation to flare up. Attempt to get 7-9 hours of restful sleep each night.

5. **Avoid Toxins:** Reduce exposure to environmental toxins by cleaning the air inside and selecting housekeeping goods wisely.

6. "Maintain a Healthy Weight": If you are overweight, try to lose weight by eating well and working out.

7. Complements: Take into account dietary supplements with anti-inflammatory characteristics, including omega-3 fatty acids, curcumin (found in turmeric), and vitamin D.

**Final Thoughts**

In order to achieve wellness, it is essential to comprehend inflammation and how it affects health. While acute inflammation is a helpful reaction to wounds and infections, persistent inflammation may be a factor in a variety of health problems, including autoimmune disorders and heart disease. We may decrease inflammation, enhance general health, and live better lives by recognizing and treating the sources of inflammation and altering our lifestyles. For a healthier, more energetic future, it is within our ability to take care of our bodies and lessen the impact of chronic inflammation.

**1.2 What is an Anti-Inflammatory Diet?**

The significance of a balanced diet must be addressed in a society where chronic diseases are on the increase, and many of us lead more sedentary lives. However, a healthy diet may have a big influence on your general health and well-being in addition to merely aiding in weight reduction. The anti-inflammatory diet is one such diet that has received a lot of attention lately. We'll examine the idea of an anti-inflammatory diet in this article, learning what it is, how it functions, and why it's thought to be a useful strategy for achieving improved health.

**Learning About Inflammation**

Understanding inflammation is essential before talking about an anti-inflammatory diet. When your body fights off infections and recovers from injuries, inflammation is a normal reaction that takes place. Your body employs this defense system to heal damaged tissue and ward off invading pathogens like bacteria and viruses. You need this acute, transient inflammation to survive.

However, when inflammation persists, issues might develop. Long after the immediate danger has passed, inflammation may continue and cause a variety of health problems. Chronic inflammation is linked to a lot of diseases, like Alzheimer's, heart disease, cancer, diabetes, arthritis, and even diabetes. In essence, it's a smoldering fire that might eventually cause harm to your body.

**Diet against Inflammation**

The anti-inflammatory diet is intended to assist in reducing this persistent inflammation. It isn't a set diet with strict guidelines but rather a method of eating that emphasizes foods that are known to lessen inflammation while avoiding those that can make it worse. This diet seeks to make your body's pro-inflammatory and anti-inflammatory substances more evenly distributed.

**Important Elements of a Diet to Reduce Inflammation**

1. **Fruits and Vegetables**: Fruits and vegetables are the foundation of an anti-inflammatory diet. They include plenty of antioxidants, vitamins, and minerals that may help reduce inflammation. These meals are a great option for anyone trying to maintain a healthy weight since they have few calories and a lot of fiber.

2. **Healthy Fats**: The anti-inflammatory diet must include unsaturated fats, which may be found in foods like olive oil, avocados, and fatty fish (such as salmon and mackerel). Omega-3 fatty acids, which are present in these lipids, are powerful anti-inflammatory compounds.

3. **Lean Protein**: Lean protein sources, such as chicken, tofu, and beans, may help lower the consumption of pro-inflammatory saturated fats that are commonly present in red meat.

4. Whole Grains: Whole Whole wheat, quinoa, and brown rice are all good sources of fiber and other nutrients. In addition, they have a lower glycemic index, which may aid in reducing inflammation and blood sugar.

5. **Spices and Herbs**: Some Spices and herbs, like ginger, turmeric, and garlic, have long been recognized for their ability to reduce inflammation. Your meals become more flavorful and healthier thanks to them.

6. **Nuts and Seeds**: Chia, flax, and walnut seeds are loaded with vitamins, minerals, and heart-healthy lipids. Additionally, they're excellent for meeting your desires for snacks without turning to processed, harmful alternatives.

7. **Fatty Fish**: Omega-3-rich fatty fish may assist in lowering inflammation and support heart health.

## Foods to stay away from

1. Sugars: Too much sugar, particularly refined sugars like those found in many processed meals, may cause inflammation and other health issues. You must limit your sugar consumption.

2. **Trans Fats**: These fats, which are often present in fried and baked items, have been directly related to inflammation and are to be avoided or restricted.

3. **Processed Foods**: Many processed foods are heavy in artificial sweeteners, harmful fats, and sugars. These foods may make inflammation worse.

4. **Red Meat**: Lean cuts of red meat should be chosen if you want to eat red meat; however, it may be a healthy addition to a balanced diet.

5. **Excess Alcohol**: Drinking alcohol excessively might cause chronic inflammation and other health problems. For optimal outcomes, use alcohol moderately or not at all.

## What Science Says

Science supports the anti-inflammatory diet theory. According to research, those who follow this eating pattern have reduced blood levels of inflammatory indicators. For instance, when an anti-inflammatory diet is followed, C-reactive protein (CRP), a measure of inflammation, tends to decrease.

Additionally, the anti-inflammatory diet is comparable to well-known healthy eating styles like the Mediterranean diet. This overlap supports the notion that maintaining overall health is equally as important as lowering inflammation.

## The Advantages of a Diet that Reduces Inflammation

Changing to an anti-inflammatory diet may enhance your health in a number of ways:

1. **Reduced chance of Chronic Diseases**: You may lessen your chance of acquiring illnesses, including heart disease, diabetes, and certain cancers, by lowering chronic inflammation.

2. **Improved Joint Health**: An anti-inflammatory diet may assist those with inflammatory joint disorders like arthritis to feel less pain and stiffness.

3. **Better Weight Management**: Eating food that is full of fruits, veggies, and lean meats will help you maintain a healthy weight, which lowers your risk of inflammation brought on by obesity.

4. **Enhanced Mental Health**: Recent studies point to the potential benefits of an anti-inflammatory diet on mood and cognitive performance.

5. **Gut Health**: A balanced gut microbiota, which is increasingly connected to inflammation and general health, may be supported by a nutritious diet.

In conclusion, a flexible and evidence-based strategy for enhancing your health by lowering chronic inflammation is an anti-inflammatory diet. You may get a variety of advantages by putting an emphasis on complete, natural meals and avoiding processed and harmful alternatives. Before making drastic changes to your eating habits, it is essential to speak with a healthcare practitioner, as with any big nutritional change. But by following this eating strategy, you may actively contribute to lowering inflammation and fostering a healthier, more energetic way of life.

## 1.3 Benefits of an Anti-Inflammatory Diet

Chronic inflammation has become a widespread health problem in today's fast-paced environment. It's a low-grade, systemic inflammation that often goes unseen but has a significant negative influence on our health; it's more than simply the occasional redness and swelling we feel when we get hurt. The good news is that by consciously choosing the things you consume, you can take charge of your health. It is now generally known that an anti-inflammatory diet full of whole, healthy foods may lower inflammation and enhance general well-being. We'll look at the various advantages of eating anti-inflammatory foods in this post.

## 1. Reduction of Chronic Inflammation

A major selling point of anti-inflammatory diets is their ability to reduce chronic inflammation. This nutrient-dense diet includes fruits, vegetables, whole grains, lean meats, and healthy fats. The fight against inflammation relies heavily on the enzymes, minerals, and vitamins included in these meals. Fish high in omega-3 fatty acids, such as salmon and mackerel, and fatty foods like walnuts and olive oil are excellent dietary sources. Omega-3 fatty acids' ability to reduce systemic inflammation is well-documented. Incorporating these foods into your diet may boost your cells' anti-inflammatory capabilities.

## 2. Promotes Heart Health

The beneficial effects of an anti-inflammatory diet on cardiovascular health are among its main advantages. Chronic inflammation raises the risk of heart disease and may damage blood arteries. This diet helps to improve blood vessel health and lowers the risk of heart-related problems by lowering inflammation. Heart disease is less likely when heart-healthy foods like avocados, berries, and almonds are consumed because they help control blood pressure and cholesterol levels.

## 3. Promotes Weight Management

The key to total well-being is to maintain a healthy weight. Emphasizing whole, fiber-rich meals helps with weight control in an anti-inflammatory diet. These foods reduce overeating by prolonging your sensation of fullness. Additionally, by lowering inflammation, this diet enhances insulin sensitivity and metabolism, making it simpler to control your weight properly.

## 4. Maintains Blood Sugar Balance

A diet that reduces inflammation may benefit those with diabetes or at risk of developing the disease. Maintaining healthy blood sugar levels emphasizes a diet rich in fibre, complex carbohydrates, and lean proteins. A decreased chance of developing type 2 diabetes is associated with stable blood sugar levels. You can maintain healthy blood sugar levels with some meals that lower inflammation and insulin resistance.

## 5. Improves Digestive Health

A diet that reduces inflammation is good for your gut health, which is important for your overall health. Having a lot of fiber-rich foods in your diet can help you have normal bowel movements, lower your risk of stomach illnesses, and feed healthy gut bacteria. Eating foods like yogurt and fermented veggies that are high in probiotics can help keep the bacteria in your gut in balance. This makes digestion and vitamin intake better.

## 6. Enhances Mental Health

Chronic inflammation has been associated with several neurological disorders, including Alzheimer's disease and cognitive decline. The anti-inflammatory diet improves cognitive function by emphasising vitamin and nutrient-packed meals and omega-3 fatty acids. These items enhance brain function, shield brain cells from damage, and decrease the likelihood of age-related cognitive decline.

### 7. Fights joint pain and arthritis

When it comes to arthritis, which is marked by inflammation of the joints, an anti-inflammatory diet could be helpful. Berry and dark leafy green vegetables, which are high in antioxidants, help the body battle oxidative stress in the joints. Arthritic pain and stiffness may be alleviated by consuming omega-3 fatty acids, which are present in fatty fish and flaxseeds.

### 8. Enhances Skin Health

Reducing inflammation may result in healthier, more vibrant skin since your skin is a reflection of your entire health. Acne, eczema, and psoriasis may all be controlled with the anti-inflammatory diet's abundance of antioxidants and good fats. These vitamins and minerals aid in skin restoration, reduce inflammation and redness, and encourage a brighter complexion.

### 9. Encourages Healthy Aging

Although aging is a natural process, you may age more gracefully by eating anti-inflammatory foods. This diet may improve your quality of life as you age by lowering inflammation and guarding against age-related disorders. By lowering the risk of chronic diseases and age-related health problems, it encourages lifespan.

### 10. Increases Immunity

The immune system is a very important part of the body's fight against getting sick. By supplying vital vitamins and minerals that promote immune function, an anti-inflammatory diet may help you have a stronger immune system. Antioxidant-rich foods, such as citrus fruits and leafy greens, improve your body's resistance to disease.

In conclusion, an anti-inflammatory diet has several advantages outside only lowering inflammation. By choosing healthier foods, you may strengthen your immune system, age gracefully, support digestive health, support brain health, improve heart health, maintain a healthy weight, balance blood sugar, support digestive health, and support brain health. It's a nutritional strategy that may make you feel better all around and help you live a longer, healthier life. Think about adding anti-inflammatory foods to your diet to get all the health and wellness benefits.

**1.4 Key Principles of Anti-Inflammatory Diet**

Inflammation due to lifestyle choices is a major health concern, and anti-inflammatory diets are gaining popularity. Many long-term diseases, including diabetes, cardiovascular disease, and arthritis, are rooted in chronic inflammation; this diet aims to reduce it. Individuals may protect themselves against inflammation-related illnesses by adhering to the principles of an anti-inflammatory diet. This article will discuss the fundamentals of an anti-inflammatory diet, including which foods exacerbate inflammation and alleviate it.

**How to Understand Inflammation**

It's critical to comprehend what inflammation is and why it matters before diving into the anti-inflammatory diet's guiding principles. The body's natural reaction to hurt, illness, or potentially dangerous stimuli is inflammation. The healing process includes acute inflammation, such as the redness and swelling that appear around a cut or injury. However, the real issue is persistent inflammation. It is a systemic, chronic, low-level inflammation that may seriously harm the body.

Poor lifestyle decisions, such as a diet heavy in processed foods, inactivity, smoking, and high levels of stress, often lead to chronic inflammation. Chronic activation of the body's inflammatory response may result in the onset of a number of disorders. Therefore, reducing chronic inflammation and enhancing general health are the main objectives of a food that reduces inflammation.

**Important Guidelines for food that reduces inflammation:**

1. You should eat a lot of whole, raw foods. A diet that reduces inflammation is based on eating whole, raw foods. Nutrient-dense foods like fresh fruits and veggies, whole grains, lean meats, nuts, and seeds may help lower inflammation. A lot of the vitamins and minerals in these foods also help your health in general.

2. *Prioritise and use omega-3 fatty acids:* Fatty fish such as salmon, mackerel, and sardines, as well as walnuts, flaxseeds, and chia seeds, contain omega-3 fatty acids, which are potent compounds that alleviate pain. By maintaining a healthy ratio of omega-3 to omega-6 fatty acids in the body, these beneficial fats prevent the inflammatory cascade of events.

   Lowering intake of omega-6 fatty acids Omega-6 fatty acids, in contrast to omega-3 fatty acids, are mostly present in dietary oils, such as maize and soybean oil. Overconsumption could lead to inflammation. Reduce your intake of processed and fried meals if you care about your health.

3. *Color Your Plate:* Fruits and vegetables' brilliant hues are a sign of their high antioxidant, vitamin, and mineral content. You may get a wide range of anti-inflammatory chemicals by including a wide array of colored fruit in your meals.

5. Be sure to choose lean protein. Chicken, fish, tofu, beans, and lentils are all good sources of lean protein. These options have less saturated fat and may lower the chance of getting diseases that are linked to inflammation.

6. Fewer refined starches should be eaten. Refined carbs are found in foods like white bread, sweet cereals, and desserts. They may raise blood sugar and cause inflammation. For a good source of carbs, choose whole grains like brown rice, quinoa, and whole wheat bread.

7. *Keep drinking water:* Water is very important for your health in general. Toxins and waste are flushed out of the body's cells more quickly and efficiently when you stay properly hydrated. Green tea is a natural drink that is high in vitamins and helps reduce inflammation.

8. *Add some heat:* Turmeric, ginger, cinnamon, and garlic are just a few of the herbs and spices that work very well to reduce inflammation. Adding these spices to your food will make it taste better and be better for you.

9. *Stay away from trans fats:* Trans fats are well-known inflammatory factors and are often present in partly hydrogenated oils. Pay close attention to food labels and avoid foods that contain these unhealthy fats.

10. *Cut down on added sugars:* Consuming too much sugar may result in obesity, which is a major cause of inflammation. A diet that reduces inflammation must exclude sugary drinks, sweets, and snacks.

11. *Exercise Portion Control:* Eating too much of anything, including nutritious meals, may cause inflammation. Always listen to your hunger cues and watch your meal amounts.

12. *Cooking techniques that reduce inflammation:* It matters how you prepare your meals. Choose cooking techniques that help preserve the nutritious content of your food, such as steaming, grilling, or baking. Do not deep fry or chargrill food since these methods may generate dangerous substances.

**Benefits of a Diet that Reduces Inflammation:**

Numerous health advantages may result from adhering to the anti-inflammatory diet's guiding principles. It lowers the risk of chronic illnesses while also enhancing general health. Among the advantages are:

- *Lower chance of developing heart disease:* A decreased risk of cardiovascular disease may be achieved via lowering blood pressure and cholesterol using an anti-inflammatory diet.

- *Better joint health* It helps lessen joint pain and stiffness, which can help control the symptoms of arthritis.

- *Improved mental well-being:* Anti-inflammatory foods may benefit mood and cognitive performance, according to certain research.

- *Weight control:* Obesity, a disorder linked to chronic inflammation, may be prevented and supported by an anti-inflammatory diet.

- *Normal blood sugar levels:* This diet is advantageous for people with diabetes since it emphasizes Low-glycemic foods may help keep blood sugar levels steady.

Finally, adhering to the fundamental tenets of an anti-inflammatory diet may enable people to take charge of their health. One may lessen chronic inflammation, decrease their risk of illness, and live a happier, more energetic life by emphasizing whole, unprocessed foods and making educated eating decisions. Although eating is just one factor in the equation, it is a strong and practical instrument for enhancing well-being and encouraging lifespan.

## 1.5 Anti Inflammatory Foods to Include in Diet

A natural and vital component of our body's protection, inflammation serves as a shield against damage and infection. Chronic inflammation, however, may result in a number of medical conditions, including cancer, autoimmune diseases, heart disease, and diabetes. The good news is that by making intelligent dietary decisions, you may have a substantial influence on your inflammatory response. In this post, we'll look at a variety of anti-inflammatory foods you may eat to lower inflammation and improve your general health.

7. *One:* "Fatty Fish" Salmon, mackerel, sardines, and trout are examples of fatty fish rich in omega-3 fatty acids, particularly EPA and DHA. The anti-inflammatory properties of these essential oils are rather powerful. Inflammation indicators

and the likelihood of developing chronic diseases may be reduced by consuming fatty fish. Add fatty fish to your diet at least twice or thrice weekly.

8. *Finally, berries:* Berries like blueberries, strawberries, and raspberries are full of antioxidants that fight inflammation, such as quercetin and anthocyanins. In addition, they have a lot of fiber, which helps keep blood sugar levels in check. Berries are good for you and taste great. Put some in your yogurt, cereal, or drink in the morning.

9. *Greens with leaves:* Lots of antioxidants, vitamins, and minerals can be found in leafy greens like spinach, kale, Swiss chard, and more. Also, they are a great source of fiber. Because they have so many of these nutrients, leafy greens are a great way to reduce inflammation and avoid the diseases that come with it. Use them in soups, salads, or stir-fries to get the most out of them.

10. *This is turmeric.* Turmeric has a bright yellow spice called curcumin that does the work. One of the best known benefits of curcumin is that it can help reduce inflammation. It may help reduce inflammation at the molecular level. Try adding turmeric to soups, stews, or curries to get the health benefits that can come from it.

11. *Nuts:* Flaxseed, walnuts, and other nuts are great sources of fiber, healthy fats, and vitamins. They have been shown to reduce inflammation in the past and may be good for your health in general. Snack on a handful of nuts or add them to soups and yogurt for a crunchy touch.

12. *Olive oil:* Olive oil from the extra virgin variety is an important part of the Mediterranean diet and is known to help lower inflammation. It has a lot of polyunsaturated fats and an antioxidant called oleocanthal. To dress salads or sprinkle over cooked veggies, use extra virgin olive oil instead of other cooking oils.

13. *Tomatillos:* Lycopene, an antioxidant with anti-inflammatory properties, is abundant in tomatoes. Consider adding tomato sauce or sun-dried tomatoes to your recipes, as cooking tomatoes releases more lycopene. They boost taste and have powerful anti-inflammatory properties.

**Eight.** Ginger Another spice that has been used for ages for its therapeutic effects is ginger. It includes bioactive substances with antioxidant and anti-inflammatory properties. You may flavor your food with dried ginger or use fresh ginger in smoothies, drinks, and stir-fries.

10. Green Tea: The polyphenols included in green tea have been demonstrated to combat cell damage and decrease inflammation. It's a tasty and hydrating way to add anti-inflammatory ingredients to your diet. Make drinking green tea a habit instead of sweetened drinks.

11. *Dark chocolate:* 10. Yes, you read it right: dark chocolate may be a component of a diet that reduces inflammation. Antioxidants abound in dark chocolate with a high cocoa content. It has been linked to less inflammatory response and enhanced heart health. Eat a little piece of dark chocolate now and then as a pleasure.

12. Vegetables and fruits come in at number eleven. A diet rich in colourful fruits and vegetables provides a wealth of antioxidants, vitamins, and minerals. Strive for a diverse array of phytonutrients if you want to get the advantages of their anti-inflammatory properties.

13. *Spicy foods:* Other spices with anti-inflammatory qualities include cinnamon, cloves, and garlic, in addition to turmeric and ginger. You may add these spices to your meals for taste and health advantages.

14. *Whole Grains*: Oats, quinoa, and brown rice are examples of whole grains that are great sources of fiber and have anti-inflammatory properties. They also assist in controlling blood sugar levels. Replace processed grains in your meals with whole grains.

15. *Beans:* Black beans, kidney beans, and lentils are just a few of the legumes that are high in fiber and antioxidants. They have a reputation for lowering the risk of chronic illnesses and reducing inflammation. Include beans in salads, stews, and soups.

16. *Foods Rich in Probiotics* A strong gut microbiota, which is essential for controlling inflammation, is supported by probiotics. The probiotics found in yogurt, kefir, sauerkraut, and kimchi are all very good for you. They help maintain a healthy and anti-inflammatory stomach by being a part of your diet.

You don't have to make big changes to your diet right away to include these foods that help reduce inflammation.Gradual changes may result in enduring habits and long-term health advantages. Try out various dishes and cooking techniques to see which ones suit you the best. A balanced diet full of whole foods serves as the cornerstone of an anti-inflammatory eating strategy, so keep that in mind. Your body will appreciate your efforts with less inflammation and enhanced general health.

Chapter 2: Breakfast Recipes

- **Recipe 1: Anti-Inflammatory Smoothie**

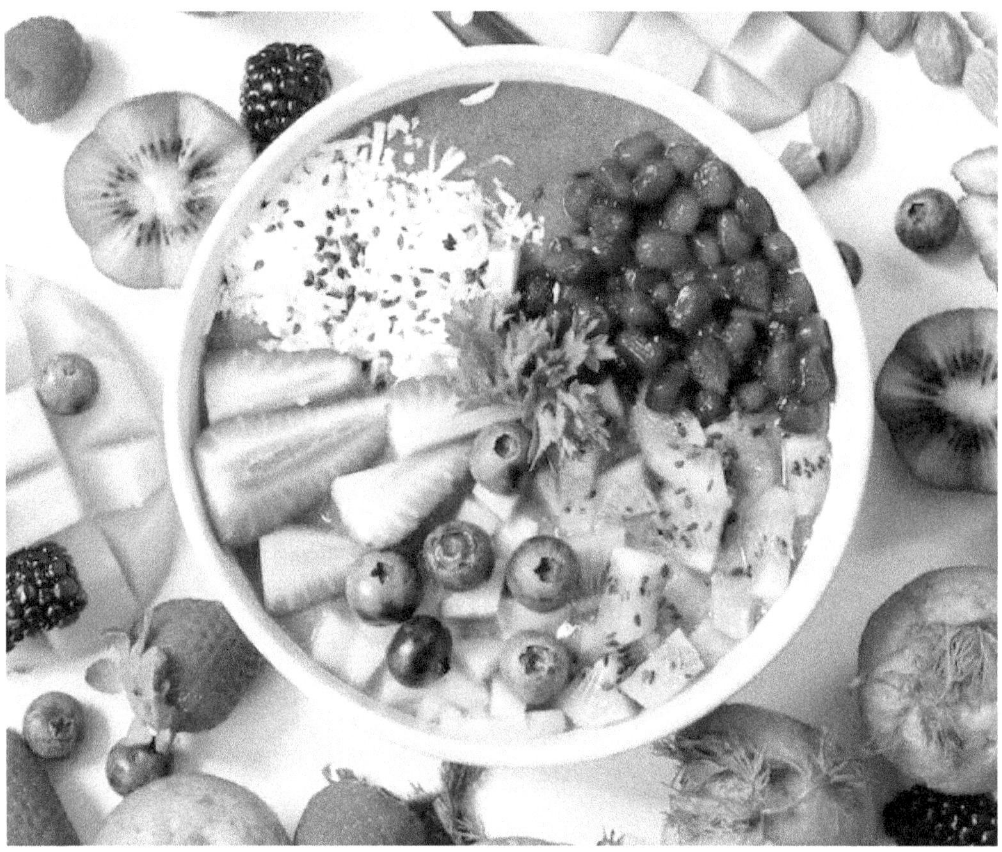

**Ingredients:**

- One teaspoon of turmeric, either whole or ground

- One teaspoon of ginger that has just been grated

- 1 cup (freezing or fresh) grapes spinach

- Half a cup of pineapple pieces, either fresh or frozen

- Half a cup of blueberries, either fresh or frozen

- Chia seeds, one tablespoon

- Ground flaxseeds: 1 teaspoon

- Half a cup of plain, low-fat, or dairy-free Greek yoghurt

- One cup of almond milk that isn't sweetened

- 1–2 teaspoons of maple syrup or honey (more is always welcome)

- 1/2 cup (for thickness, if you want) ice chunks

**Instructions:**

If using fresh leaves, properly wash the spinach before using it. Put the pineapple chunks, blueberries, and almond milk in the freezer for around 30 minutes before mixing if you want a cooler smoothie.

**Ingredients:**

Blend the Greek yogurt, almond milk, spinach, pineapple, blueberries, chia seeds, grated ginger, and turmeric in a blender. At this point, add honey or maple syrup if you want your smoothie to be sweeter.

Starting on low and gradually increasing the speed will get the blender to high speed. Stir until combined. Blend the smoothie ingredients until they form a thick and velvety mixture. To thin down the mixture, add some ice cubes and stir.

Test the smoothie's flavor and make any adjustments. Add extra honey or maple syrup if you'd like it to be sweeter, and mix for a little while to combine.

If you like a thicker, spoonable consistency, pour the anti-inflammatory smoothie into a glass or a bowl before serving. A few blueberries, a fresh pineapple slice, or some chia seeds may be used as decorations.

*Enjoy:* Drink your anti-inflammatory smoothie carefully and enjoy the mouthwatering taste combination. Along with being loaded with anti-inflammatory components, this nutrient-dense smoothie also offers a delicious and refreshing method to boost your health and well-being.

**Cooking Notes:**

You are free to change the component amounts to suit your preferred level of flavor. You may increase the amount of ginger or turmeric if you like a stronger taste. The sweetness may also be changed by increasing the amount of honey or maple syrup.

This smoothie is simple to modify if you must adhere to dietary restrictions. Use a plant-based yogurt like almond or coconut yogurt for a dairy-free alternative. To limit additional sugars, ensure the almond milk you choose is unsweetened.

Be careful when using turmeric since it may stain surfaces and clothes. You should mop up spills right away and put on an apron.

This smoothie serves as a flexible foundation for further customization. You may use anti-inflammatory components like a handful of kale, a fresh lemon slice, or a scoop of collagen powder for more protein.

In addition to being tasty, this anti-inflammatory smoothie is a wholesome method to boost your health. A reviving and fulfilling beverage made with turmeric, ginger, spinach, and other healthy ingredients may be enjoyed for breakfast, a snack, or refreshment after exercise. It's a wonderful supplement to your anti-inflammatory diet.

- **Recipe 2: Turmeric and Ginger Overnight Oats**

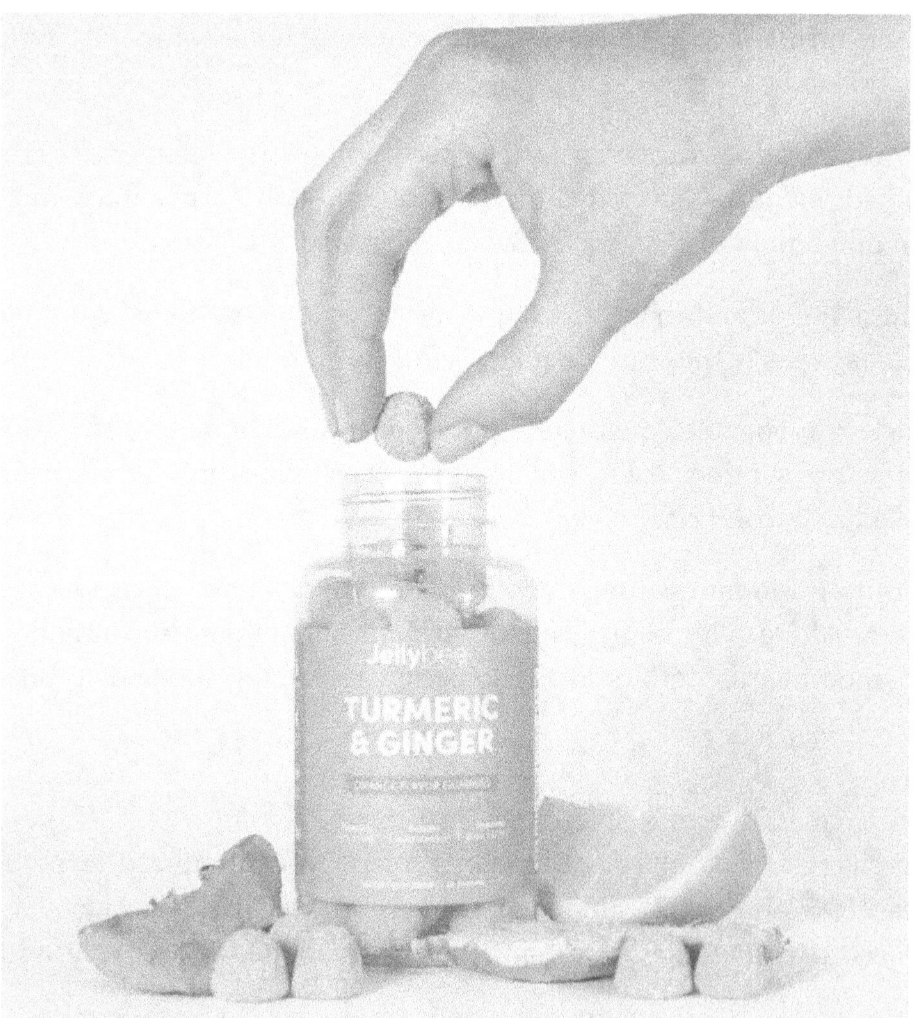


**Ingredients:**

*Oats Rolled:* 1/2 cup.

- 1 cup milk, no matter what kind it is

- Half a teaspoon of turmeric powder

- One tablespoon of ginger that has been sliced or chopped very small

- 1 to 2 teaspoons of honey or maple syrup (adjust the amount of sweetness you want)

- Try adding half a teaspoon of ground cinnamon for an extra cinnamon kick.

- One tablespoon of chia seeds (optional; adds thickness)

- Fresh Berries: 1/2 cup (your choice of blueberries, strawberries, raspberries)

- Two tablespoons of chopped nuts (almonds, walnuts, or pecans for topping)

- 1/4 cup Greek yogurt (optional; for creaminess)

- 1/2 teaspoon (optional; for taste) vanilla extract

- Add a little salt to improve the taste.

**Instructions:**

Get the ingredients ready: Grate or finely chop the fresh ginger first. Before shredding the ginger, you may take the skin off using the back of a spoon. Measure each of the other ingredients.

***Dry ingredients:*** Combine the rolled oats, ground turmeric, ground cinnamon (if using), and a dash of salt in a bowl or other overnight oats-friendly container. Your overnight oats' foundation will be made of these dry components.

After adding the almond milk, grate or chop the ginger and add it to the list of wet ingredients. At this point, you may add honey or maple syrup if you want your oats sweeter. Add a little bit of vanilla essence for added taste.

***Optional Additions:*** You may add chia seeds to your overnight oats to increase their nutritious worth. They'll add fiber and healthy fats to the mixture and thicken it.

***Mix Everything Well:*** Stir Everything together until it is well mixed. For the turmeric to contribute its vivid color and anti-inflammatory qualities, ensure it is dispersed evenly.

Refrigerate your container by covering it with plastic wrap or a lid. It should be kept in the fridge for at least four hours, preferably all night. As a result, the oats may absorb the liquid and become creamy and soft.

Remove the oats from the fridge first thing in the morning or at your leisure when you are ready to consume them. Give everything a good stir, and ask, "Too thick?" if the consistency is too thick. Cream it up again by adding a little more almond milk.

*Add Toppings:* Add fresh berries to the turmeric and ginger overnight oats. Excellent choices include raspberries, strawberries, and blueberries. Top with chopped nuts like pecans, walnuts, or almonds for more texture and crunch.

*Optional Creaminess:* If you want your oatmeal to have a creamier texture, top it with Greek yogurt. It increases the protein level and also gives the dish more creaminess.

*Drizzle with Honey:* To increase sweetness and presentation, you may drizzle some more honey or maple syrup on top.

*Enjoy:* With a spoon, enjoy the taste and health advantages of your homemade turmeric and ginger overnight oats. This wholesome meal is a wonderful way to start the day with some anti-inflammatory goodies.

**Cooking Notes:**

Add more or less. You can use honey or maple syrup if you like. The sweetness is too strong.

If you don't like how grated ginger feels in your mouth, you may squeeze out the juice using a fine sieve or cheesecloth and flavor the oats.

To make your overnight oats even more interesting, try experimenting with various toppings and add-ins like sliced bananas, shredded coconut, or dried fruits.

Remember that the oats will grow softer the longer you leave them in the refrigerator. To get the oat texture you desire, adjust the soaking time.

A tasty and healthy way to start the day is with these overnight oats with turmeric and ginger. The warming effects of ginger, the anti-inflammatory properties of turmeric, and the creamy texture of oats provide a filling breakfast that is not only tasty but also full of health benefits. Take pleasure in this filling meal as part of your pain relief plan diet.

- **How to Make It 3: Avocado and Tomato Breakfast Salad**

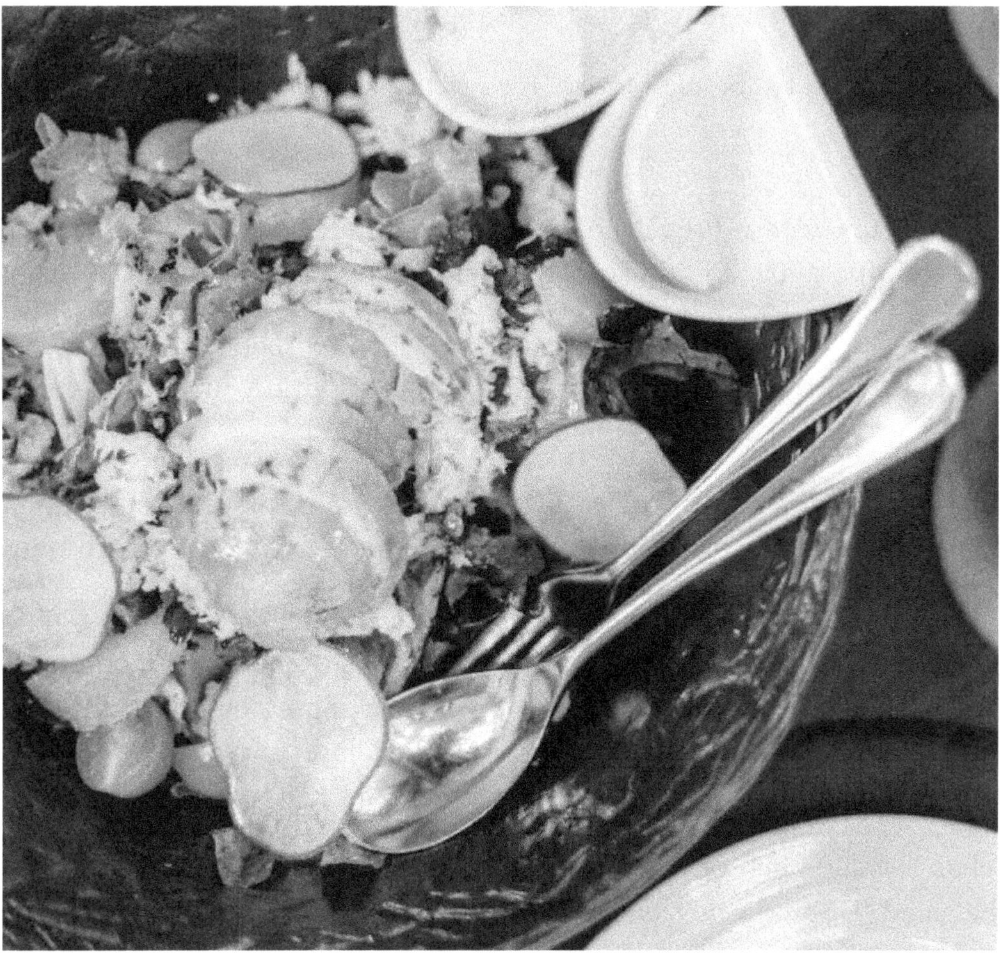

## Ingredients:

**Avocado:** 1 ripe avocado, chopped after being peeled and pitted.

- 1 or 2 medium-sized to large tomatoes, cut up

- Small diced red onion, 1/4 cup

- Snipped basil leaves, 1/4 cup

- Two tablespoons of lemon juice, or about one lemon.

**Olive Oil Extra Virgin:** 2 Tablespoons

- To taste, add 1/2 teaspoon of salt.

- For a little additional heat, add 1/4 teaspoon of black pepper.

- 1/4 cup of crumbled feta cheese is not required but makes it taste better.

- 2, sliced or quartered hard-boiled eggs (optional, for added protein)

- Slices of toasted baguette or bread: for serving (optional)

**Instructions:**

*Get the ingredients ready:* Prepare all of your components first. Slice the red onion thinly, dice the ripe avocado and tomatoes, and slice the fresh basil leaves — slice or quarter hard-boiled eggs now if you decide to add them.

Make the sauce by combining the lemon juice and extra virgin olive oil in a small bowl. The salad will get a spicy kick from this simple sauce.

*Combine the ingredients:* Put the diced avocado, tomatoes, finely sliced red onion, and chopped basil leaves in a large bowl. These ingredients' vivid hues and invigorating fragrances will make your salad aesthetically attractive.

*Dressing:* Drizzle the avocado, tomato, onion, and basil with the lemon and olive oil dressing. To ensure that the dressing covers all the ingredients equally, gently mix everything. In addition to flavoring the avocado, the lemon juice also helps keep it from turning brown.

You can change how much salt and black pepper you use to suit your taste before you season the salad. Do not forget that adding a little salt could make the tomatoes and avocado taste much better.

*Optional Additions:* Top the salad with crumbled feta cheese if you want more taste and nutrition. The fresh ingredients taste delicious with the feta's creamy, salty overtones.

Distribute the avocado and tomato breakfast salad among separate bowls or plates to be served. Serve it with toasted bread or baguette pieces on the side if you like a heartier breakfast.

Hard-boiled eggs may be used as a typical breakfast garnish or an additional protein boost. Hard-boiled eggs can be sliced or cut into quarters.

Enjoy the flavorful fusion of fresh basil, lemon zest, and tomatoes that are luscious and creamy with avocado. In addition to being a feast for the senses, the salad is a healthy way to start the day.

**Cooking Notes:**

Prepare the salad before serving to preserve the avocado's freshness and color. To avoid the avocado from browning, if you need to prepare it beforehand, refrigerate it separately and add it just before serving.

You may alter this morning's salad by adding extra cucumber, bell peppers, or olives to fit your preferences.

Leave out the optional feta cheese and hard-boiled eggs for a vegan variation. To create new taste combinations, try experimenting with other herbs, such as mint, parsley, or cilantro.

Start your day with this delicious and nutritious Avocado and Tomato Breakfast Salad. It's a fantastic choice for anybody trying to reduce inflammation in their diet since it's full of beneficial nutrients and has avocado's rich, creamy texture. This salad is perfect for breakfast alone or as a side dish with other breakfast items.

- **Recipe 4: Chia Seed Pudding with Berries**

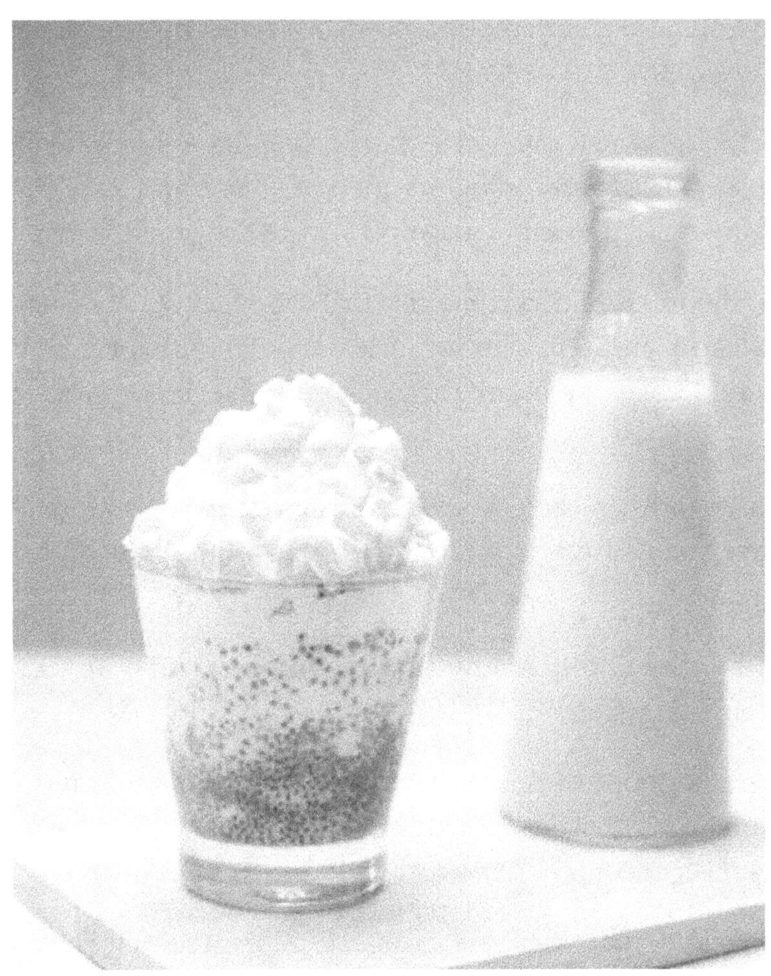

**Ingredients:**

**Seeds of chia:** 1/4 cup

- There should be one cup of milk. You can use soy milk, almond milk, coconut milk, or any other kind of milk you like.

- 2 to 3 tablespoons of honey or maple syrup (adjust the amount of sweetness you want)

- Half a teaspoon of vanilla extract

- You can have blueberries, strawberries, raspberries, or a mix of these: 1/2 cup.

- 6 to 8 fresh mint leaves (optional garnish)

**Instructions:**

Chia Seeds with Liquid: Combine the chia seeds with the milk of your choice (such as almond milk) in a mixing dish. Make sure the chia seeds are uniformly dispersed in the liquid by stirring the mixture well.

Add honey or maple syrup for sweetness and a dash of vanilla essence for flavor to sweeten and flavor the dish. To properly integrate the sweetener and vanilla, stir the mixture once more. To get the right amount of sweetness, taste the combination.

*Cover and refrigerate:* Put the mixture in a container that won't let air in or use plastic wrap to cover the bowl. Keep it in the fridge for at least four hours, or better yet, all night. Because of this, the chia seeds might soak up the liquid and become pudding-like.

*Stir and Inspect:* Once the liquid has cooled down, stir it well. There's more pudding because the chia seeds have swelled up. Is it too thick? Add a little milk and mix it in until it's the right consistency.

Put the pudding together by dividing it among serving dishes or cups. To display the lovely layers, use transparent glasses or jars.

*Add Mixed Berries:* A liberal amount of mixed berries should be placed on each dish. Use any mix of your preferred berries, including blueberries, strawberries, and raspberries. This brings a splash of color and a sweet flavor.

Add a few fresh mint leaves to the servings as a garnish (optional) for a lively and fresh touch. Mint enhances the aesthetics and enhances the taste of the berries.

Chia seed pudding with berries tastes best when served cold. Please take a delicious and wholesome breakfast, snack, or dessert.

**Cooking Notes:**

Chia seed pudding may be made in a variety of ways. Sliced bananas, chopped almonds, coconut flakes, or a dab of nut butter are just a few toppings and flavors you may try.

You may change the sweetness to your liking by varying the honey or maple syrup. You may also swap out sweeteners like agave nectar or stevia if preferred.

Before adding the berries, add a dollop of yogurt or coconut yogurt to the pudding to increase its creaminess.

Scaling up this recipe is simple. You may double or triple the components to make many servings for a party or meal preparation.

Chia seed pudding is an easy make-ahead alternative since it can be kept in the fridge for 3–4 days.

A tasty and wholesome treat, Chia Seed Pudding with Berries is excellent for breakfast or as a light dessert. Chia seeds, milk, and sweet berries combine to make a delicious and aesthetically pleasing meal. This pudding is a lovely compliment to any anti-inflammatory meal, whether consumed as a hydrating breakfast or a guilt-free treat.

- **Recipe 5: Breakfast Bowl with Quinoa**

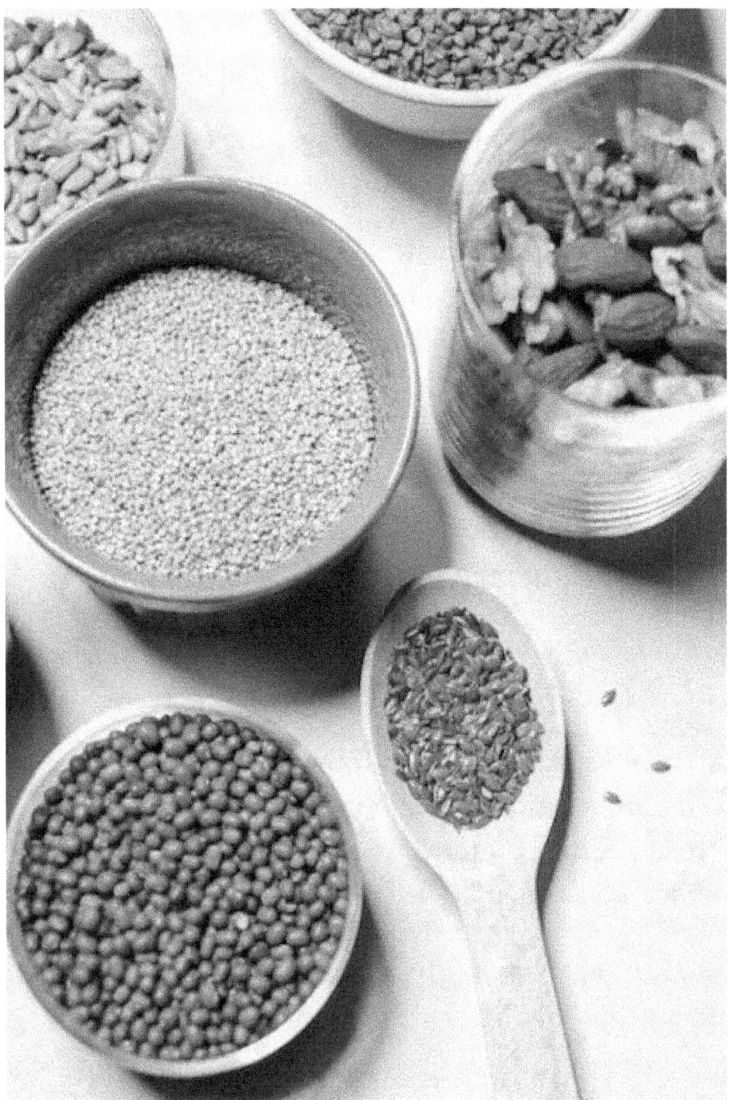

## Ingredients:

- 1 cup of Quinoa Milk (not cooked): 2 cups of milk of your choice, such as cow, almond, soy, or any other kind.

- 2 to 3 tablespoons of honey or maple syrup (adjust the amount of sweetness you want)

- One teaspoon of vanilla extract

**Cinnamon, ground:** 1/2 teaspoon

- Fresh Fruit: 1 cup (apples, berries, bananas, or any other fruit you choose, chopped)

- 1/4 cup of nuts and seeds (either chia seeds, chopped walnuts, or sliced almonds)

- 1/2 cup Greek yogurt (optional to make it creamier)

- 1/4 cup of chopped apricots, raisins, or figs, if you want.

**Fresh mint leaves:** Decorative (optional) garnish

**Instructions:**

Rinse quinoa well under cold running water before cooking to remove harsh flavours. Combine the quinoa and two cups of milk in a medium-sized saucepan. Over high heat, bring the mixture to a boil.

Once boiling, reduce heat to simmer, cover, and continue cooking. Cook the quinoa for 15–20 minutes on low heat or until most of the water has been absorbed. Things will never stick if you stir them constantly.

*After cooking the Quinoa:*

1. Please take it off the heat and add something tasty.

2. Add ground cinnamon for a cozy, soothing scent, vanilla essence for flavor, and honey or maple syrup for sweetness.

3. Make the sweetness as sweet as you want.

*Prepare Fresh Fruit:* Prepare your fresh fruit while the Quinoa slightly cools. Depending on your desire, you may cube apples, wash berries, or cut bananas into slices.

Build the breakfast bowl by dividing the cooked and sweetened Quinoa among serving dishes. Choose your favorite fresh fruit, nuts, or seeds to garnish each dish. This results in a mix of color and texture.

Greek yogurt may be added (optionally) if you want the Quinoa and fruit to have more creaminess and protein. This creates a delicious texture and taste contrast.

*Include Dried Fruit (Optional):* Add dried fruit like raisins, cranberries, or chopped apricots for sweetness and a chewy texture.

Add a few fresh mint leaves to each bowl for a fragrant and revitalizing finishing touch.

Quinoa breakfast bowls are best consumed right away while they are still warm. Enjoy the mellow combination of nutty Quinoa, sweet fruit, and cozy spices.

***Cooking Notes:***

Please put your favorite fruits, nuts, and seeds in your breakfast dish to make it uniquely yours. Sliced peaches, chopped mango, or even a dusting of coconut flakes are optional additions.

To change the taste profile of your quinoa breakfast bowl, try experimenting with other spices like nutmeg or cardamom.

To get the desired consistency, change the milk's volume. Add milk while cooking or just before serving if you like a creamier texture.

You can make this breakfast dish vegan by substituting maple syrup for honey and using milk from plants (almond or soy, for example).

Breakfast bowls made with Quinoa are adaptable and may be eaten warm or cold. The Quinoa may be made beforehand, and the bowls can be assembled as required.

A hearty and nutritious quinoa breakfast bowl is the perfect way to begin your day. The anti-inflammatory diet will love it for all the protein, fibre, and beneficial ingredients it contains. Eating this bowl for breakfast or as a satisfying snack will give you energy all morning, thanks to the delicious combination of flavours and textures.

Chapter 3: Appetizers and Snacks

- **Recipe 6: Roasted Red Pepper Hummus**

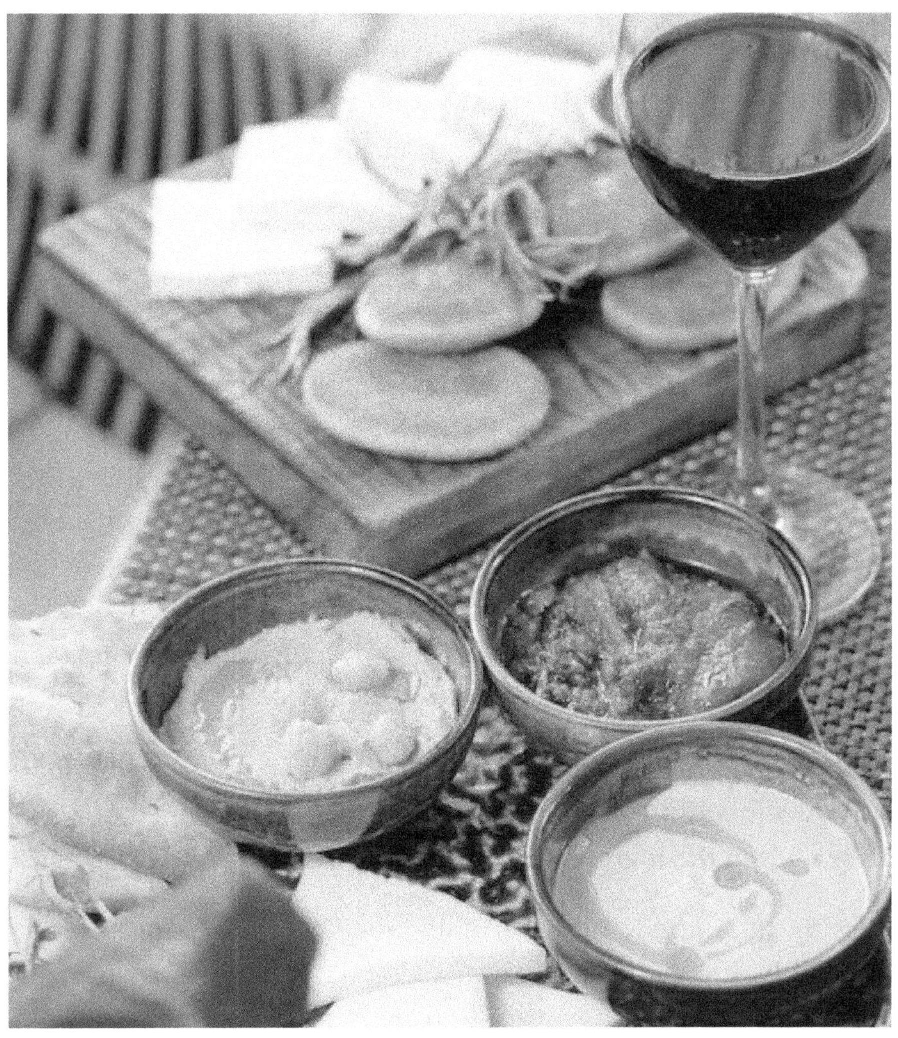

**Ingredients:**

- One can (15 ounces) of rinsed and drained chickpeas.

- One cup (about two big peppers) of roasted red peppers should be drained and dried.

- 1/4 cup (sesame paste) of tahini

- Two minced garlic cloves

**Two tablespoons of lemon juice, or about one lemon.**

**Cumin seed:** 1 teaspoon

- 1/2 teaspoon of paprika (plus more for garnish)

- If you'd want it hotter, add 1/4 teaspoon of cayenne pepper.

- 1/2 teaspoon of salt, or more if you like it.

- Approximately 2-3 tablespoons of extra-virgin olive oil (plus more for drizzling in case needed)

- 2 to 3 tablespoons of water (to make it runnier)

- For garnish, use fresh parsley.

**Instructions:**

**Get the Red Peppers Roasted:** Ensure the roasted red peppers in jars are drained and dried well before use. Settle whole red bell peppers onto a baking sheet. Brown and blacken the skins by turning the pieces over regularly in a hot broiler. Using this procedure, you can prepare meals to perfection. Put them in a sealed plastic bag and steam them for about 10 minutes after that. The skins will be simpler to peel using this method. It is recommended to wait for peppers to cool down before using them. Afterwards, remove the seeds and peel the potatoes.

**Items utilized:** Put the rinsed and drained chickpeas in a food processor with the chopped garlic, tahini, lemon juice, cumin, paprika, salt, and cayenne pepper (if using). Whisk together after adding the ingredients.

Blending or processing the ingredients in a food processor will ensure they are mixed thoroughly and smoothly. It may be necessary to scrape down the sides of the bowl and mix the ingredients again to ensure they are all properly incorporated.

To change the consistency, put the extra-virgin olive oil and water into the food processor as it works. If you add more water, the hummus might get thinner. If you add more olive oil, it might get creamier.

You should taste the hummus and make any necessary spice changes. You can make it taste better by adding more salt, lemon juice, or spices.

Move the roasted red pepper hummus to a serving bowl before you serve it and add any toppings you want. Add some extra-virgin olive oil on top to make it shine. Sprinkle some paprika on top for color, and if you like, add some fresh parsley for a burst of flavor.

*Enjoy:* You can put your own roasted red pepper hummus on sandwiches and wraps or serve it with cheese, crackers, veggie sticks, or pita bread.

**Cooking Notes:**

You may gently pinch the chickpeas between your thumb and fingertips to remove the outer skins for a creamier hummus. Despite being optional, this step might result in a smoother texture.

Play around with the tastes by experimenting with smoked paprika or ground coriander to give a touch of smokiness or earthiness.

Change the spiciness of your hummus to suit your preferences. Increase the cayenne pepper or add some red pepper flakes if you like it hot.

Any roasted red pepper hummus that is left over should be refrigerated in an airtight container. It has a week-long shelf life. Drizzle a thin coating of olive oil over the top to keep it fresh.

This Roasted Red Pepper Hummus is a tasty and colorful dip ideal for parties, picnics, or spreading on your favorite sandwiches. The combination of roasted red peppers and flavorful spices produces a lovely blend of smokiness and warmth. Enjoy this homemade hummus' rich aromas and creamy texture as a nutritious supplement to your anti-inflammatory diet.

*Hummus with Spicy Roasted Red Peppers:* Consider boosting the cayenne pepper or adding red pepper flakes to your hummus if you like spicy meals. Find your chosen amount of heat by tasting as you go.

Smoked paprika should be used instead of ordinary paprika to enhance the smoky taste. If you want an even stronger smokiness, add some liquid smoke.

*Creamy Texture:* You may peel the chickpeas before blending them if you want an extremely creamy texture. Although it takes some time, the end product is smooth hummus.

*Protein Boost:* You may add a scoop of plain Greek yogurt or a teaspoon of protein powder to the mixture to boost the amount of protein. This is a fantastic choice for those who consume a lot of protein.

*Fresh Herbs:* To add freshness and a splash of color, try using fresh herbs like basil, parsley, or cilantro. Finely slice them and mix them into the hummus.

Lemon, lime, or orange zest may be added to hummus to brighten the taste profile and give it a zesty edge.

*Serving recommendations:*

To round up your roasted red pepper hummus, serve it with pita chips, carrots, cucumbers, celery, cherry tomatoes, bell pepper strips, or pita bread.

*Hummus as a Sandwich Spread:* Use hummus as a tasty sandwich or wrap spread. Your favorite lunch preparations get a pleasant creaminess and taste boost from it.

To make a creamy salad dressing, thin the hummus with a little water or lemon juice. Grain salads, pasta salads, and salads with roasted vegetables all benefit from its use.

*Bowl Topping:* For a creamy, flavorful topping, drizzle the hummus over grain bowls, Buddha bowls, or salad bowls.

*Grilled Vegetable Dip:* For a tasty and nutritious side dish, combine hummus with grilled veggies like zucchini, eggplant, or asparagus.

**Storage Advice**

Store any extra hummus in the fridge in a jar that won't let air in. It can be kept for a week.

Consider freezing it in little pieces to extend its shelf life. It's recommended to use hummus for recipes or as a dip rather than spreading it since it could have a slightly different texture after being thawed.

**Authentic Pita Chips:**

You may quickly create pita chips at home to serve your hummus. This is how:

**Ingredients:**

- Pita bread: normal or whole wheat

- Brush with olive oil.

- Sea salt is used to season.

**Instructions:**

Heat the oven to 375 degrees Fahrenheit (190 degrees Celsius).

The best way to cut pita bread is into triangles or wedges.

Ensure that each bread slice faces up before placing it on a baking pan.

The pita pieces should be rubbed with olive oil and sea salt.

To prepare the pita chips for baking, preheat the oven. To get a golden brown and crisp outside, bake them for 8 to 10 minutes.

Allow them to cool after removing them from the oven. Enjoy the roasted red pepper hummus without the pita chips!

- **Recipe 7: Cucumber and Greek Yogurt Dip**

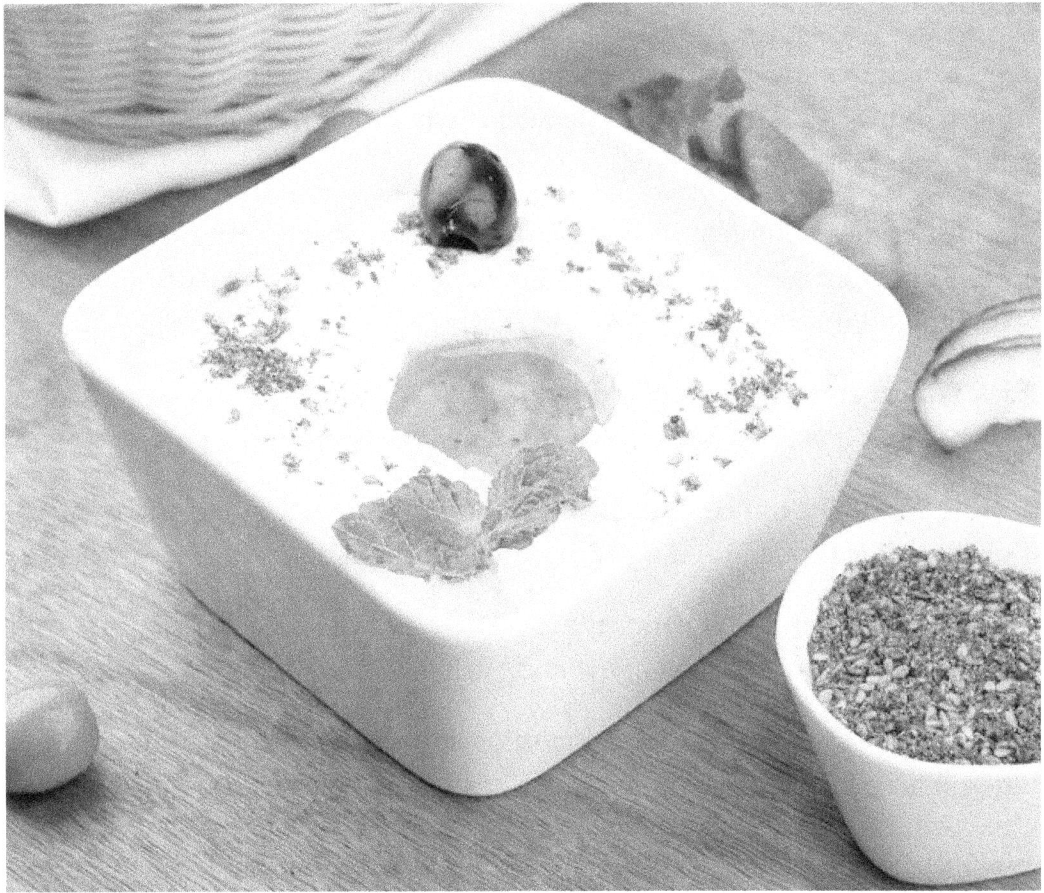

**Ingredients:**

Greek yogurt: 1 cup (full-fat or reduced-fat, if desired)

**Cucumber:** Grate 1 medium cucumber after it has been peeled and seeded.

- One minced clove of garlic

- Two teaspoons of freshly chopped fresh dill

- One tablespoon of lemon juice, or about one lemon.

- Olive Oil Extra Virgin: 1 Tablespoon

- 1/2 teaspoon of salt, or more if you like it.

- For a little additional heat, add 1/4 teaspoon of black pepper.

- 1/2 teaspoon of pepper (optional for garnishing)

**Mint Leaves:** As an optional garnish

**Instructions:**

Make sure to remove the cucumber's skin before cooking it. Use a spoon to remove the seeds after halving them lengthwise; discard them. Grate the cucumber into tiny pieces using a box grater or food processor.

After shredding the cucumber, drain it in a fine-mesh strainer or a fresh kitchen towel. To keep the dip from getting overly watery, squeeze away any extra liquid. Drain the cucumber, then set it aside.

The Greek yogurt should be prepared by being placed in a mixing basin. Greek yogurt is popular because it is thick and creamy, making it perfect for dipping.

*Garlic, minced:* Finely mince one clove of garlic. For a smoother texture, use a garlic press. Stir the garlic flavor into the yogurt after adding it.

To add fresh dill, carefully chop the herb to unleash its fragrant fragrance. Stir thoroughly after adding it to the yogurt and garlic combination.

*Add Lemon Juice:* To make one tablespoon of lemon juice, squeeze the juice from one lemon. It will give the yogurt combination a zesty and sour kick if you add it.

*Integrate Grated Cucumber:* Gently blend the yogurt mixture with the finely grated, drained cucumber. The cucumber will give the dip a cool, crisp texture.

*Salt and Pepper to Taste:* With the dip, season with salt and black pepper as desired. Add a little at a time and adjust the quantity as required.

Extra-virgin olive oil should be drizzled over the dip's surface. This not only improves the appearance but also provides a rich taste.

*Optional garnishes:* Add a pinch of paprika for an additional splash of color and flavor. Fresh mint leaves provide a pleasant garnish.

Put the dip in the fridge for at least 30 minutes before covering it and serving. By letting the ingredients mix, cooling makes the taste better.

*Serve and Take Note:* With various dippers, such as pita bread, pita chips, carrot sticks, cucumber slices, celery sticks, or bell pepper strips, serve your cucumber and Greek yogurt dip.

**Cooking Notes:**

You may add another minced clove of garlic for a greater garlic taste.

Try experimenting with various herbs and spices to personalize the dip. Additions like fresh parsley, chives, or cayenne pepper may be delicious.

Add a spoonful of mayonnaise or sour cream to the dip to make it creamier.

Add some milk or extra virgin olive oil if you want the dip to be lighter.

Any extra dip should be put in the fridge in a container that won't let air in. It will stay good for a few days, but the texture may get a little thinner over time as the cucumber releases water. Before serving, mix everything well.

An energizing and healthful choice, this cucumber and Greek yogurt dip is ideal for gatherings, picnics, or a quick snack. A wonderfully creamy and refreshing dip combines aromatic herbs, crisp cucumber, and creamy Greek yogurt. Enjoy it with your preferred sides as a dip, spread, or sauce.

- **Recipe 8: Spiced Almonds**

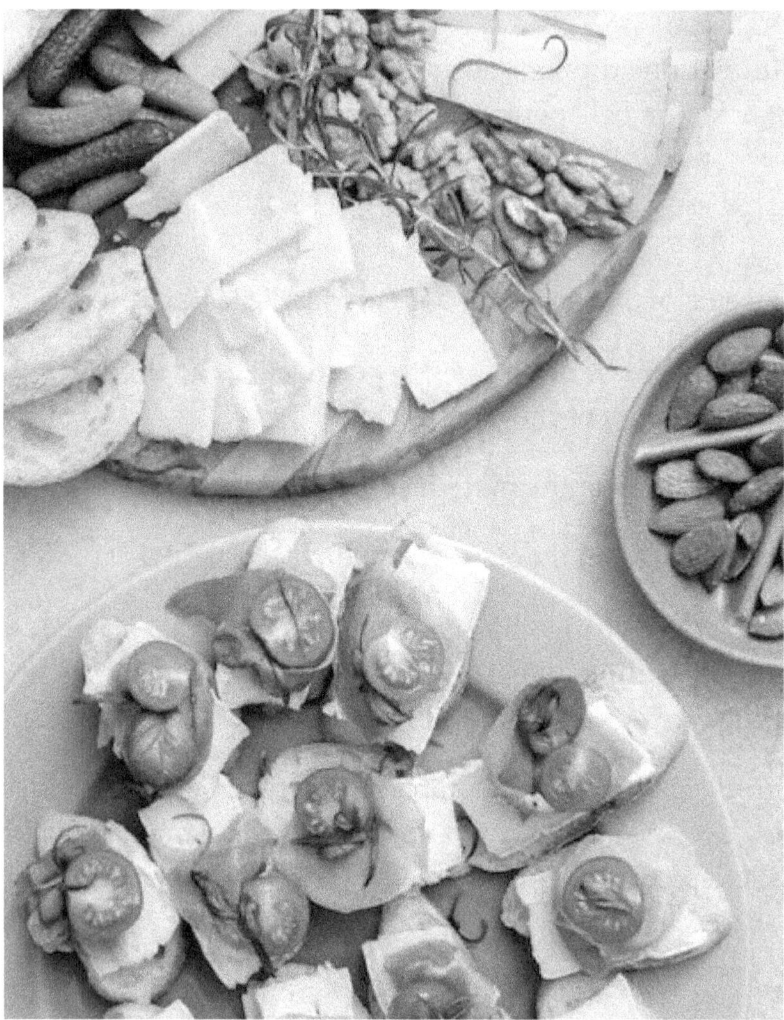

**Ingredients:**

- 2 cups of raw, unsalted almonds

- One tablespoon of olive oil

- **Cumin seed:** 1 teaspoon

**Paprika ground:** half a teaspoon

- 1/4 teaspoon of ground cayenne pepper (adjust for spiciness)

- Cinnamon-ground: 1/4 teaspoon

- 0.5 teaspoon salt (adjust to taste)

- One tablespoon of honey (optional, for a hint of sweetness)

## Instructions:

Preheat the oven to 175 Fahrenheit (350 Celsius). Parchment paper or silicone baking mats line a baking sheet for easy cleaning.

Prepare the raw, unsalted almonds in a large mixing basin.

*Olive Oil:* Pour the olive oil over the nuts. The spices will stay better, and the almonds will have a lovely roasted flavour.

*Add Spices:* Season the almonds with salt, ground cumin, paprika, ground cayenne pepper, and ground cinnamon. Your almonds will get complexity, warmth, and a tinge of spice from these spices. At this point, you may add honey if you'd like a little sweetness.

*Toss and coat:* Mix the almonds with the oil and spices slowly, either with a spoon or your hands, until they are well covered. Make sure that the spice is spread out evenly among the nuts.

Spread the seasoned almonds equally on the baking sheet that has been preheated. To achieve consistent roasting, Try to put them all on top of each other.

*Roast in the Oven:* Roast the almonds on a baking sheet for 12–15 minutes or until they develop a nutty aroma and a deeper shade of brown. In the final five minutes, be careful not to let them brown too much by watching them.

*Complete Cooling:* After taking the spiced almonds out of the oven, cool them on the baking sheet. As they cool down, they will keep becoming crisper.

You may enjoy the spiced almonds as a snack or appetizer when they've cooled completely, or you can keep them in the fridge for later. They may be kept fresh for up to two weeks if sealed in an airtight container and kept at room temperature.

## Cooking Notes:

You can adjust the heat level to your preference. If you want a milder taste, Cayenne pepper may be eliminated or reduced in quantity. On the other hand, if you like spicy treats, add a little extra cayenne.

Honey may be used with the spiced almonds if you want both sweet and salty tastes. While roasting, the honey will caramelize, providing a delicious contrast to the spices.

Add flavors and spices like smoked paprika, chili powder, or garlic powder to produce several iterations of spiced almonds.

To keep the almonds crunch, let them cool fully before storing them. They could get softer if they are kept while still warm.

These seasoned almonds make a delicious snack and are a flexible addition to salads, yogurt toppings, charcuterie, and cheese boards.

- **Recipe 9: Zucchini Fritters**

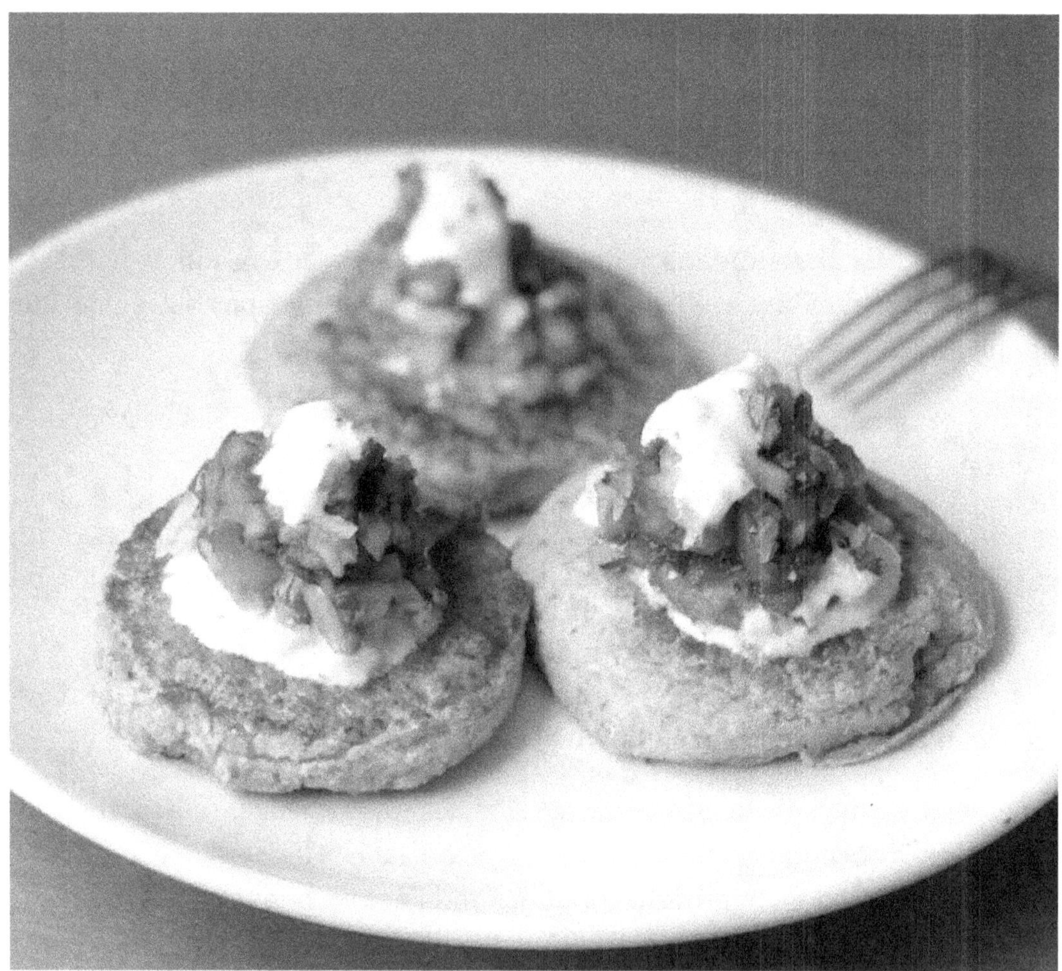

**Ingredients:**

- Two medium-sized zucchini, grated, equals roughly 2 cups.

- One teaspoon salt

- one huge egg

- 1 and a half cups of regular flour

- Grate 1/4 cup of Parmesan cheese.

- Two teaspoons of chopped herbs that are just picked (parsley, dill, or basil are all good options)

- Could you please chop one clove of garlic?

- 1/4 teaspoon black pepper, or more if you like it spicier

- Two to three teaspoons of olive oil

- For serving, use sour cream or Greek yogurt.

- Lemon wedges: An optional garnish

**Instructions:**

Start by shredding the zucchini using a box grater or a food processor's grating attachment. Then, season the grated zucchini with salt. Grated zucchini should be in a fine-mesh sieve or a fresh kitchen towel. One teaspoon of salt should be added, and the food should rest for 10 to 15 minutes. This will assist in draining the zucchini of extra moisture.

*Squeeze Out Extra Moisture:* After the zucchini has rested, squeeze out as much moisture as possible using your hands or a kitchen towel. How much liquid can be eliminated will amaze you. To avoid soggy cakes, ensure the zucchini is as dry as possible.

Whisk the egg in a mixing basin to combine with the batter. Incorporate the strained and minced zucchini, all-purpose flour, shredded Parmesan cheese, sliced garlic, and chopped fresh herbs. All of the components must be well combined. The batter must be sufficiently thick to maintain its form.

Heat a large frying pan or skillet over medium-low heat with a few drops of olive oil until hot. Get the oil to the bottom of the pan.

Drop spoonfuls of zucchini batter into the hot oil to make patties. Press down on each piece using the back of the spoon to make a cake. Three to four minutes on each side, or until golden and crisp, is the recommended cooking time for the cakes. Whether or not you need to work in batches depends on the size of your pan.

After removing the cakes from the pan, place them on a tray to soak up any remaining oil. Place paper towels on top. They keep working after going through this process.

Fried zucchini is at its most delicious when served hot. Squeeze some fresh lemon juice on top and top with a spoonful of sour cream or Greek yoghurt to make them even more flavorful.

**Cooking Notes:**

With the seasoning, you can get creative. Add a dash of smoked paprika for a smokey taste or a sprinkle of cayenne pepper for extra spice.

If you'd like to make these cakes gluten-free, you may substitute almond flour for all-purpose flour or use gluten-free flour or a gluten-free mix.

Try experimenting with various plants. Popular options include fresh parsley, dill, and basil, but you may also use other herbs, such as chives or cilantro, depending on your tastes.

For a satisfyingly crispy surface, ensure your skillet or frying pan is hot before adding the patties.

Zucchini fritters that are left over may be kept in the fridge for a day or two. To keep them crisp, reheat them in a preheated or toaster oven.

The crisp, light taste of zucchini may be enjoyed in pleasing amounts in zucchini fritters. These cakes are fantastic as appetizers, side dishes, or even a light dinner when paired with a side salad. They're a preferred option for adding extra zucchini throughout the summer because of their adaptability and delectable flavor.

- **Recipe 10: Stuffed Bell Peppers**

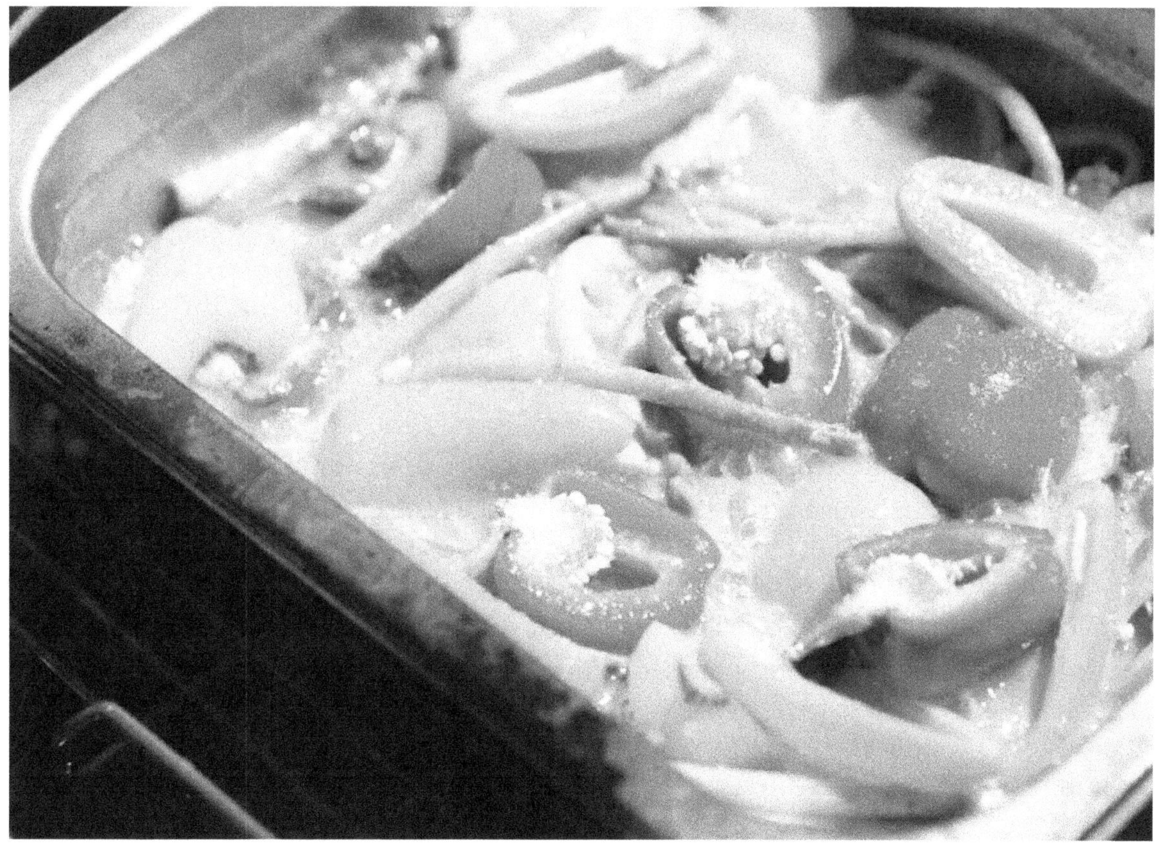

**Ingredients:**

*Bell peppers:* 4 big, any color bell peppers

For vegetarians, a pound of ground beef or turkey, or 2 pounds of ground chicken or crumbled plant-based protein.

White, brown, or a combination of both cups of cooked Rice

One medium onion, finely chopped

Two minced garlic cloves

One can of tomato sauce, about 14 ounces

Tomatoes, diced: 1 can (14 ounces)

Italian seasoning, measuring one teaspoon

To taste, add 1/2 teaspoon of salt.

For a little additional heat, add 1/4 teaspoon of black pepper.

One cup of cheese shreds (mozzarella, cheddar, or any other cheese you like).

For garnish, use fresh parsley or basil.

**Instructions:**

Warm up. Warm the oven up to 190 degrees Celsius (375 degrees Fahrenheit).

To get the peppers ready, carefully cut off the tops and take out the seeds and skins. If the peppers don't stand up straight, cut a little off the bottom to make the surface smooth. Peppers that are hollow should be put away.

*Cook the Rice:* Prepare it according to the box's directions, then put it aside. White or brown Rice may be used, depending on your desire.

*Cooking the Ground Meat:*Brown the ground turkey or beef in a large skillet over medium-high heat. Till the colour becomes pinkish-brown, use a spatula to mash it while it cooks so it crumbles evenly. When necessary, trim off any excess fat.

*Sauté onion and garlic:* Place the minced and finely diced onion in the same pan. The onion should be sautéed for two to three minutes until transparent and aromatic.

**Combine beef and Rice:**

1.  Put the onions, garlic, and cooked ground beef in the pan.

2.  To the bowl, add the cooked rice and diced tomatoes.

3.  Sprinkle the Italian spice, salt, and pepper on top.

All of the ingredients should be well mixed. Let the flavors boil for approximately 5 minutes to allow them to blend.

*Tomato Sauce Addition:* Add the tomato sauce to the meat and rice, and then stir it all together. Let the mixture cook on low heat for five more minutes so it can thicken slowly.

*Bell Pepper Stuffing:* Carefully fill each bell pepper with the meat and rice mixture, gently pushing it down to ensure it is well-packed. You may fill them out.

Once they're on a serving platter, bake them. Cover the dish with foil and place it in the oven. The peppers should be tender after 30–40 minutes in the oven. You may bake softer peppers for a little longer if you want softer peppers.

***Add Cheese:*** Once the paper is removed, top each whole pepper with shredded cheese. Please place them in the oven after 5 to 10 minutes or when the cheese bubbles and melts and the edges brown.

Add some fresh parsley or basil to the stuffed bell peppers after taking them out of the oven to give them color and some life. Please serve hot.

**Cooking Notes:**

Add items like sliced mushrooms, chopped spinach, or corn to the filling to enhance taste and nutrients.

Replace the ground beef in this recipe with plant-based crumbles or additional veggies like chopped mushrooms or zucchini to make it vegetarian.

For various taste characteristics, try using cheeses other than parmesan, feta, or pepper jack as a topping.

Leftover bell peppers with stuffing taste great. Peppers that are left over can be kept in the fridge for a few days in a container that doesn't let air in.

Any filling left over may be used as the foundation for a delectable pasta sauce or eaten by itself as a substantial rice and beef meal.

A traditional and substantial meal, stuffed bell peppers mix the sweetness of bell peppers with savory and delicious stuffing. This dish provides a well-balanced mix of grains, veggies, and protein, making it a filling and healthy dinner for any occasion. Fresh from the oven, savor the flavor and fragrance of these wonderful stuffed peppers.

# Chapter 4: Soups and Salads

- **Recipe 11: Anti-Inflammatory Broccoli Soup**

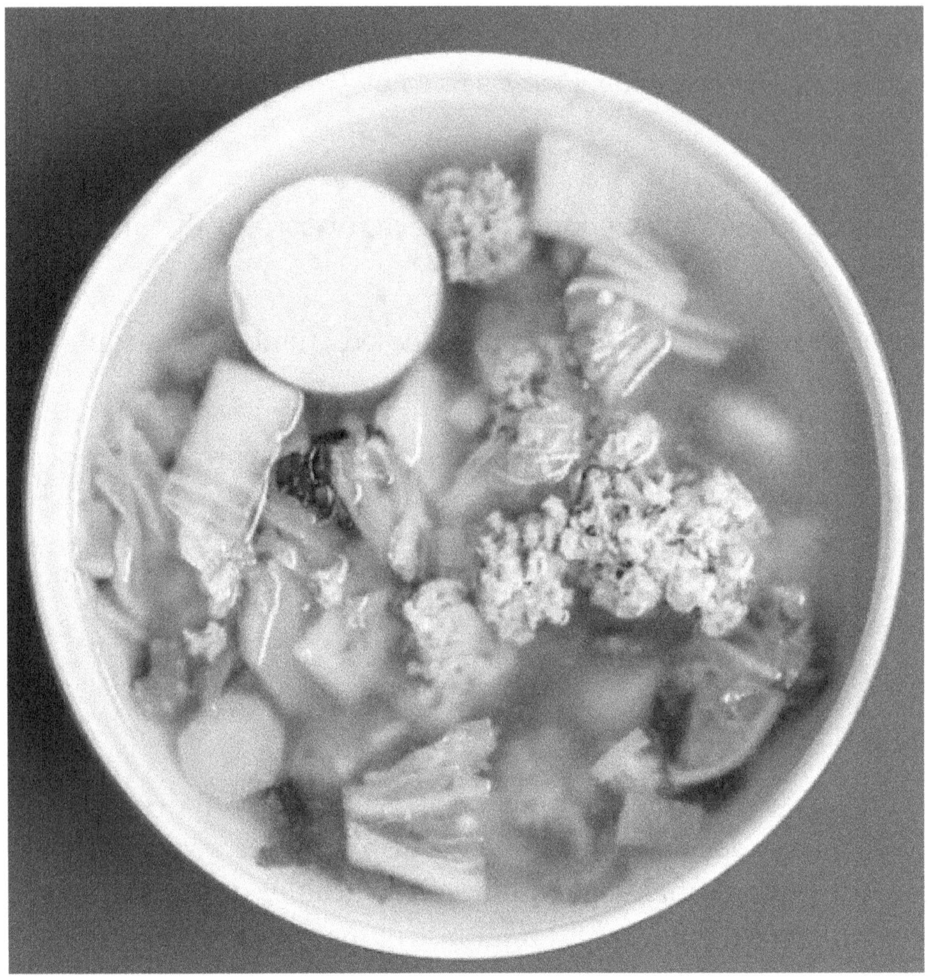

## Ingredients:

- Broccoli cut into florets, 4 cups (approximately two big heads).

- One medium-sized onion, chopped; two to three minced garlic cloves, please

- *Celery:* two sliced stalks

- Two medium-sized carrots, diced.

- Two teaspoons of olive oil

- One teaspoon of ground turmeric

- One teaspoon of freshly grated ginger

- Add half a teaspoon of black pepper, or more to taste.

- 4 cups of vegetable soup low in salt

- One cup of coconut milk, either full-fat or light, from a can

- 1/2 teaspoon of salt, or more if you like it.

- 2 tsp of lemon juice, which is about 1 lemon.

- Fresh cilantro or parsley can be used as a garnish.

**Instructions:**

*Sauté Aromatics:*

1. A big soup pot set over medium-low heat should be used to warm the olive oil.

2. Once the onion, carrots, celery, and garlic are tender, sauté them.

3. After around five to seven minutes of cooking, the veggies should be tender and the onion translucent.

***Ginger and Turmeric Should Be Added:*** Add the freshly grated ginger and the ground turmeric. These spices give the soup a taste and have anti-inflammatory properties — Sauté the ingredients for a further 2 minutes or until aromatic.

Broccoli should now be added. Stir in the chopped broccoli florets and simmer until they are brilliant green and softening.

The low-sodium vegetable broth should be added, ensuring all the veggies are completely immersed. Your soup will be built around this.

*Simmer:* First, bring the soup to a low boil. The broccoli and veggies should be soft and creamy, so cover and simmer for about 15 to 20 minutes on low heat.

Use caution when blending the soup with an immersion blender; you want it smooth and creamy. Is an immersion mixer not necessary? The soup may be gradually transferred to a standard blender. Be cautious not to develop pressure while mixing hot liquids; a little airflow is all it takes.

To mix the soup in a standard blender, cook the soup in the saucepan first. Return it to the burner and reduce the heat.

*Stir in Coconut Milk:* Add some canned coconut milk to the soup to make it smoother and bring out the rich smells of the broccoli and spices. To mix, stir it well.

*To taste, add salt and pepper.* Toss in some black pepper and salt into the soup. Add a little at a time and adjust the quantity as required.

*Add Lemon Juice:* To get roughly two tablespoons of lemon juice, squeeze the juice from one lemon. It will give the soup brightness and acidity if you add it. To integrate, stir.

*Warm Through:* After adding the coconut milk, let the soup warm over moderate heat, but avoid bringing it to a boil.

Ladle the anti-inflammatory broccoli soup into dishes before garnishing. Garnish with fresh cilantro or parsley to add color and freshness if desired.

**Cooking Notes:**

Adjust the thickness of the soup by adding additional vegetable broth or decreasing the simmering time. You may customize the thickness according to your preference.

Throw in some baby spinach or kale in the final few minutes of cooking for some more flavor and nutrition. Plus, it will wilt into the broth while providing extra nutrients. Toss in a pinch of cayenne or red pepper flakes with the aromatics as they simmer if you want your cuisine on the hotter side.

You have four days to enjoy this soup once you make it. When you're ready to enjoy it, gently reheat it in the microwave or on the stove.

Incorporate whole-grain bread or a simple salad into your anti-inflammatory broccoli soup for a satisfying and nutritious dinner.

This anti-inflammatory broccoli soup is delicious and packed with nutrients that fight inflammation. It's a bowl of pleasure that will fulfill your appetites and help your overall health. If you're searching for a filling supper or a healthy way to include more vegetables into your diet, this homemade soup will do the trick.

- **Recipe 12: Spinach and Strawberry Salad**

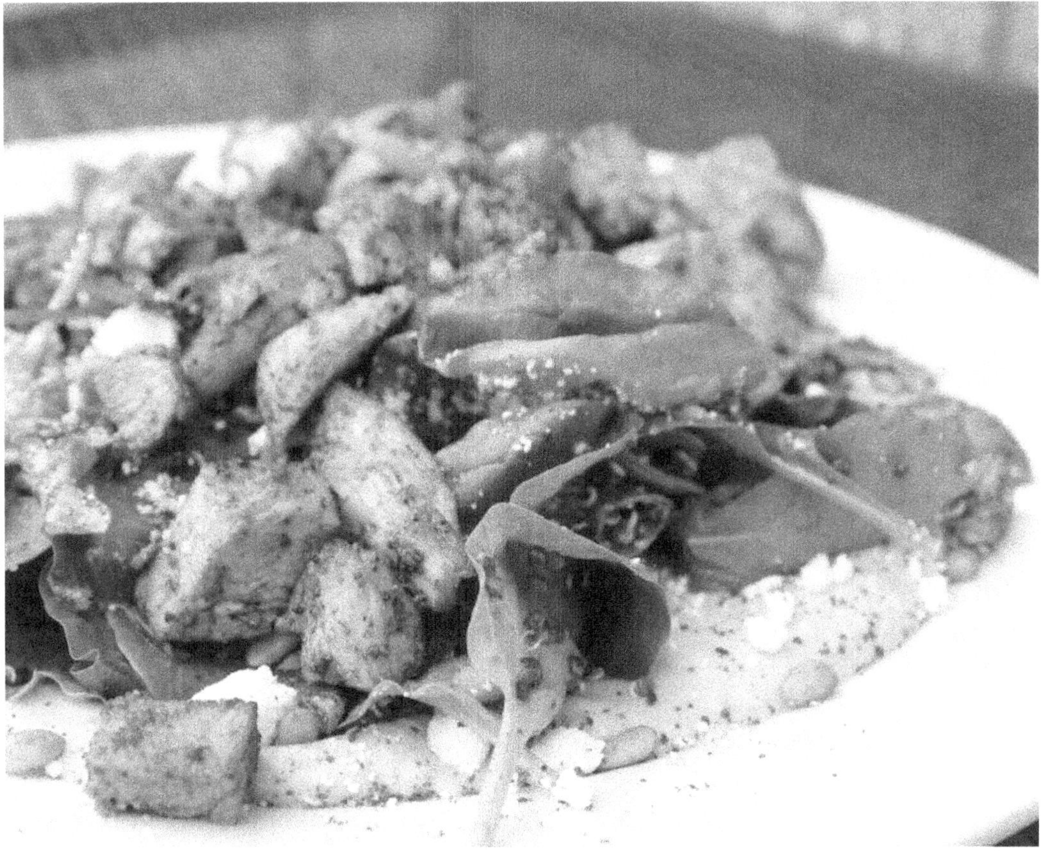

**Ingredients:**

- 6 cups of washed and dried baby spinach

- 2 cups grapes, peeled and cut into slices

- Cut one small red onion into thin slices.

- The 1/2 cup of feta cheese that has been diced is optional.

- 1/2 cup of chopped nuts (healthy options include simple roasted nuts) or nuts (walnuts or pecans with added sugar).

- 1/4 cup sauce made with balsamic vinegar (bought or made at home; see recipes below)

- For garnishing, tear or thinly slice 1/4 cup of fresh basil leaves.

- To taste, add salt and black pepper.

- Homemade Balsamic Vinaigrette Dressing:

- Vinegar: 3 teaspoons of balsamic

- Olive Oil Extra Virgin: 1/2 cup

- Mustard de Dijon: 1 teaspoon

- One tablespoon honey, or, for a vegan version, one tablespoon maple syrup

- One minced clove of garlic, please

- A quarter teaspoon of salt and a quarter teaspoon of black pepper

**Instructions:**

*For the homemade balsamic vinaigrette dressing:*

Honey (or maple syrup), chopped garlic, salt, black pepper, and Dijon mustard should all be mixed together in a small bowl.

While continuing to whisk, sprinkle in the extra virgin olive oil gradually. By emulsifying the dressing, a creamy and well-blended texture is produced.

Taste the dressing and make any necessary seasoning adjustments. You may increase the sweetness or tanginess by adding extra honey or vinegar.

Wait to add the sauce to the salad until you are ready.

*For the salad with spinach and strawberries:*

*Get the ingredients ready:* Baby spinach leaves should be washed and dried. The strawberries should be hulled before being cut into rounds. Slice the red onion very thinly. If used, coarsely cut the candied pecans or walnuts and crumble the feta cheese.

*Prepare the Salad:* Place the baby spinach, strawberry slices, red onion, and crumbled feta cheese (if using) in a large salad dish. Toss everything together carefully to combine.

*Add Nuts:* Top the salad with candied pecans or walnuts. These give the meal a lovely crunch and nutty taste. Use plain roasted nuts for a more healthful alternative.

**Dressing:**

1. Sprinkle the salad with the balsamic vinegar sauce right before you serve it.

2.  If you believe it needs extra sauce, add more after you've added a little.

3.  Give the salad a gentle toss so that the sauce covers all of the ingredients.

Any amount of salt and freshly ground pepper will work. Toss the salad and garnish it as desired. Top with shredded or thinly sliced fresh basil leaves for a verdant flavour.

*Serve and Enjoy:* As a zingy and colorful appetizer, side dish, or light supper, serve your spinach and strawberry salad immediately.

**Cooking Notes:**

You are welcome to modify this salad to suit your tastes. You may use other items like sliced almonds, goat cheese, or avocado for different textures and tastes.

Remove the feta cheese from the salad or replace it with a dairy-free substitute to make it vegan.

If you like a sweeter dressing, you may modify the honey (or maple syrup) in the balsamic vinaigrette to your preferred sweetness.

To make this salad into a filling main dish, add grilled chicken breast, tofu, or chickpeas for more protein.

This salad is best eaten right away to preserve the vegetables' freshness and the spinach's crispness.

Spinach and strawberry salad is ideal for a light and refreshing supper since it combines sweet and salty ingredients well. The brilliant colors and contrasting textures create a tasty meal that is attractive to the eyes and the taste. This dish gives a burst of freshness ideal for any occasion, whether served as a salad or a quick lunch.

- **Recipe 13: Tomato Basil Quinoa Salad**

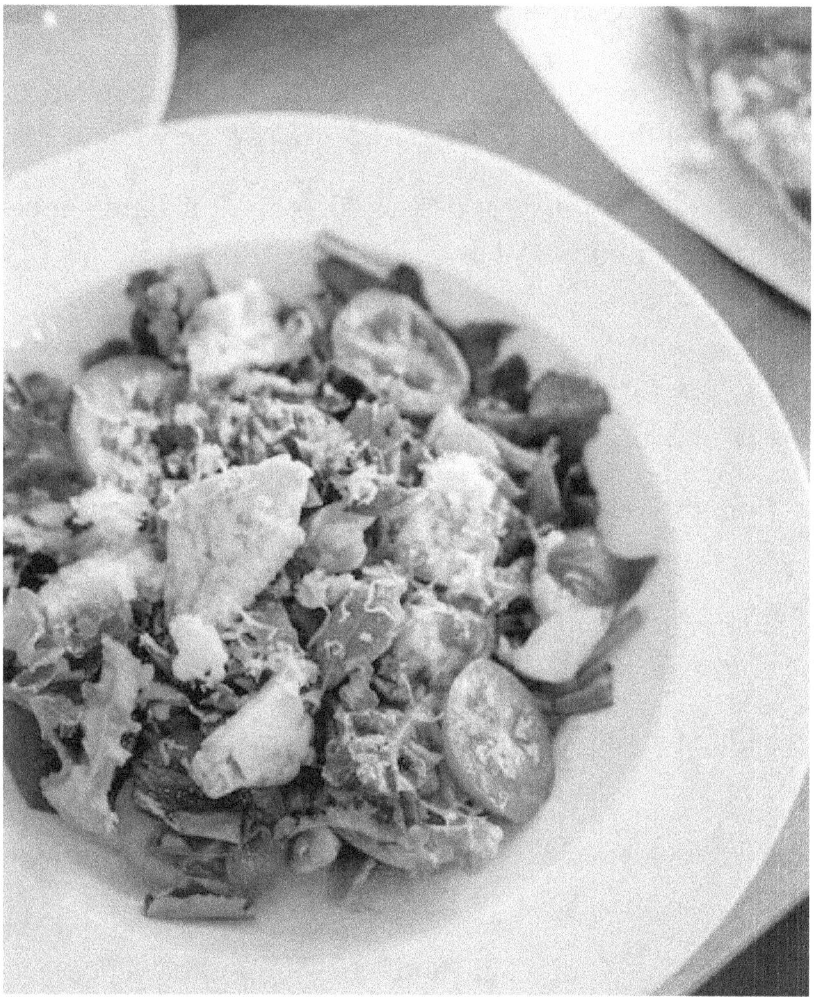

**Ingredients:**

- 1 cup (uncooked) of quinoa

- Half a pint (or around 2 cups) of cherry tomatoes.

- 1 cup of freshly cut, loosely packed fresh basil leaves

**Red onion:** 1 tiny, finely sliced red onion.

- Feel free to garnish with half a cup of kalamata olives, chopped and sliced.

- The 1/2 cup of feta cheese that has been diced is optional.

- Extra Virgin Olive Oil: 1/4 cup

- A couple of tablespoons of balsamic vinegar

- Would you want one clove of garlic minced?

- 1/2 teaspoon of salt, or more if you like it.

- For a little additional heat, add 1/4 teaspoon of black pepper.

**Instructions:**

*Cook the quinoa:* TTo remove any remaining bitterness:

1. Give the quinoa a good rinse under cold running water.

2. After washing the quinoa, add 2 cups of water to a medium-sized saucepan and bring it to a boil. The mixture should be brought to a boil over medium-high heat.

3. Bring to a boil, then decrease the heat to low and cover for around 15 minutes.

The quinoa will get softer as the water soaks into it. Once it reaches room temperature, please please take it off the heat.

Whisk together the garlic powder, balsamic vinegar, extra-virgin olive oil, salt, and pepper in a small bowl. Follow these steps to the letter to make the vinaigrette. For a salad, this is a must-have ingredient.

**Tips for Meat Preparation:** Meanwhile, finely slice the red onion, cut the cherry tomatoes in half, and split the fresh basil leaves into large parts. Set aside the quinoa to cool. If you want to add olives and crumbled feta cheese, chop them.

*Ingredients:* Toss the cooked quinoa with the chopped cherry tomatoes, red onion, fresh basil, and (if using) Kalamata olives in a big salad bowl.

To add some flair to the salad, drizzle the dressing over it. Coat the items lightly by tossing them in the sauce. The salad will be even more delicious with the dressing drizzled over it.

*Feta cheese addition (optional):* Now, crush the feta cheese over the salad. The contrast between the other ingredients and the creamy, acidic feta is excellent.

Taste the salad and make any necessary spice adjustments. If desired, you may increase the amount of salt, black pepper, or olive oil.

Refrigerate the salad for at least 30 minutes before serving it covered. The tastes might combine while cooling, increasing the taste in general.Put the salad in the fridge for at least 30 minutes before covering it and serving it. As it cools, the tastes may blend together, making the overall taste better.

Add more fresh basil leaves as a garnish before serving to add color and a herbaceous scent to the tomato basil quinoa salad.

**Cooking Notes:**

Feel free to add your ingredients to this salad to make it your own. You may add chopped bell peppers, cucumbers, or even some diced avocado for added freshness and texture.

Remove the feta cheese from the salad or replace it with a dairy-free substitute to make it vegan.

If you want to create a vinaigrette with a certain flavour profile, try apple cider or red wine vinegar.

If this salad is the main course, you could want to add some grilled chicken, shrimp, or chickpeas for some extra protein.

Leave Over tomato basil quinoa salad in the fridge for up to three days if it's in a container that won't let air in. You can eat it as a side dish, a quick meal, or a snack that will fill you up.

A colorful and wholesome recipe that captures the aromas of summer is tomato basil quinoa salad. The combination of fluffy quinoa, sweet cherry tomatoes, aromatic basil, and a tangy vinaigrette produces a pleasing fusion of flavors and textures. This salad is a celebration of fresh vegetables that is great for warm weather or whenever you want a clean, light dinner. It may be eaten as a meal by itself or as a cool side dish.

- **Recipe 14: Turmeric and Lentil Soup**

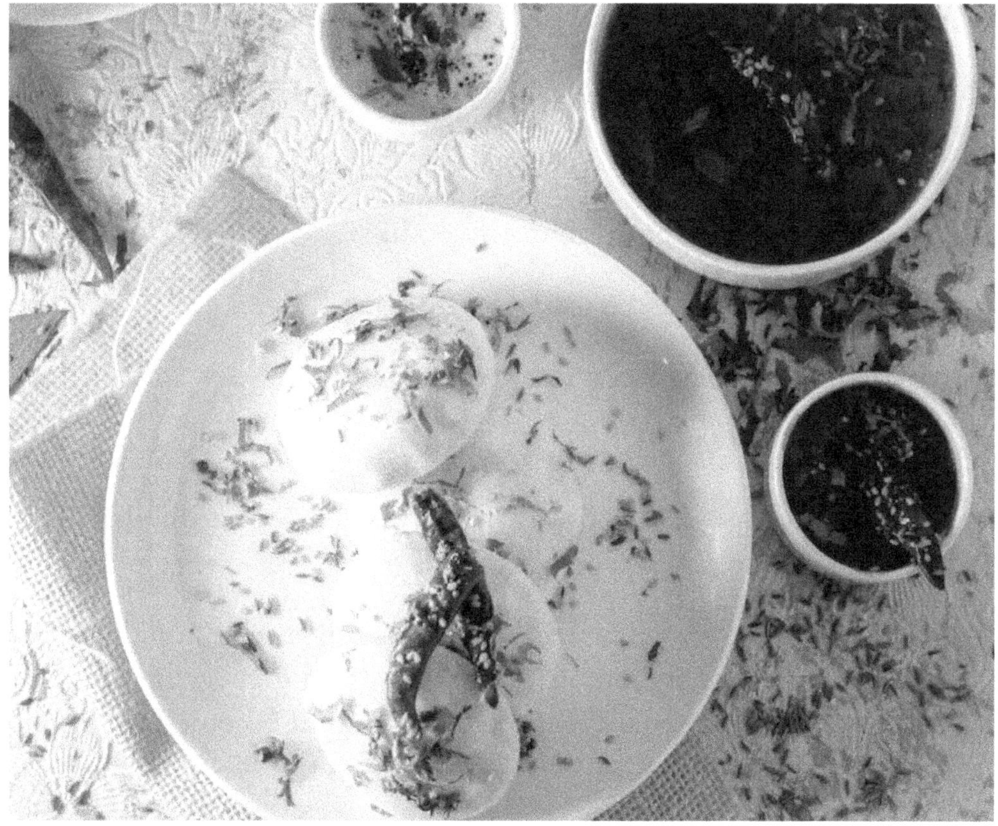

**Ingredients:**

- 1 cup dry and washed red lentils

- One medium onion, chopped

- Two medium-sized carrots diced.

- Celery: two sliced stalks

- Three to four garlic cloves cut up

- 1 inch piece of fresh ginger grate

- Turmeric, measuring half a teaspoon

- Sumatran spice, measured in teaspoons

- Ground coriander, measuring half a teaspoon

- 1/4 teaspoon cayenne pepper (adjust for spiciness)

- 8 cups of vegetable soup low in salt

- One cup of coconut milk, either full-fat or light, from a can

- 2 tsp of lemon juice, which is about 1 lemon.

- One teaspoon of salt, or as much as you like

- 1/2 teaspoon of black pepper, or more if you like

- Fresh cilantro or parsley can be used as a garnish.

- Twenty-two milliliters of extra-virgin olive oil

**Instructions:**

Fill a fine-mesh screen or sieve with cold water and pour it over the lentils. This will keep them clean. Drain them and set them aside.

Heat the extra virgin olive oil in a large saucepan over medium heat. Sauté the aromatics. Slice the carrots, celery, onion, garlic, and fresh ginger, then toss them into the skillet. The veggies should soften, and the onion should become transparent after 5 to 7 minutes of sautéing.

Combine the turmeric, coriander, cumin, and cayenne pepper powders to make the spice mixture. Warm the soup with these fragrant spices by sautéing them for 2 minutes or until they release their flavour.

Before adding rinsed red lentils to the pot, add low-sodium vegetable broth. Mix everything by stirring vigorously. The concoction has to Simmer until it comes to a boil.

Simmer: Bring the soup to a simmer over medium heat, covered, for 20 to 25 minutes, or until the veggies and lentils are cooked through.

Mash the soup: Use an immersion mixer to make it creamy and smooth. Without a mixer that can be submerged? There are a few steps to transfer the soup to a standard blender. When combining heated liquids, use caution and ensure enough air circulation to prevent pressure from building up.

To mix the soup in a standard blender, cook the soup in a saucepan first. Reduce the heat and return it to the burner.

Pour the canned coconut milk into the mixture. It will complement the lentils and spices with a touch of sweetness and smooth out the meal. Mix well by stirring.

Before serving:

1.  Add salt and black pepper to the soup according to your taste.

2.  Take a small amount at first and adjust the amount as needed. The acidity and brightness may be enhanced by adding a little lemon juice.

3.  Mix by stirring.

*Warm Through:* After adding the coconut milk, let the soup warm over moderate heat, but avoid bringing it to a boil.

*Serving and garnishing:* Put bowls of the lentil and turmeric soup in front of you. Add a splash of color and a herbal smell with fresh cilantro or parsley.

**Cooking Notes:**

Depending on your taste, add more or less cayenne pepper to the soup to make it milder or hotter.

Make careful to use canned, dairy-free coconut milk if you want to make this soup vegan.

Add chopped tomatoes, spinach, or kale for more flavor and nutrients during the last few minutes of simmering. They'll wilt into the soup and provide more flavorful layers.

Any soup that is left over should be refrigerated in an airtight container. It may be reheated on the stovetop or microwave and kept nicely for a few days.

The earthy aromas of red lentils and fragrant spices combine with turmeric's anti-inflammatory qualities to create the hearty and nourishing meal known as "turmeric and lentil soup." This recipe makes a silky, colorful soup that is both savory and healthy. Enjoy it as a hearty meal that will keep you healthy all year or as a warm bowl of comfort on a frigid day.

- **Recipe 15: Cabbage and Kale Coleslaw**

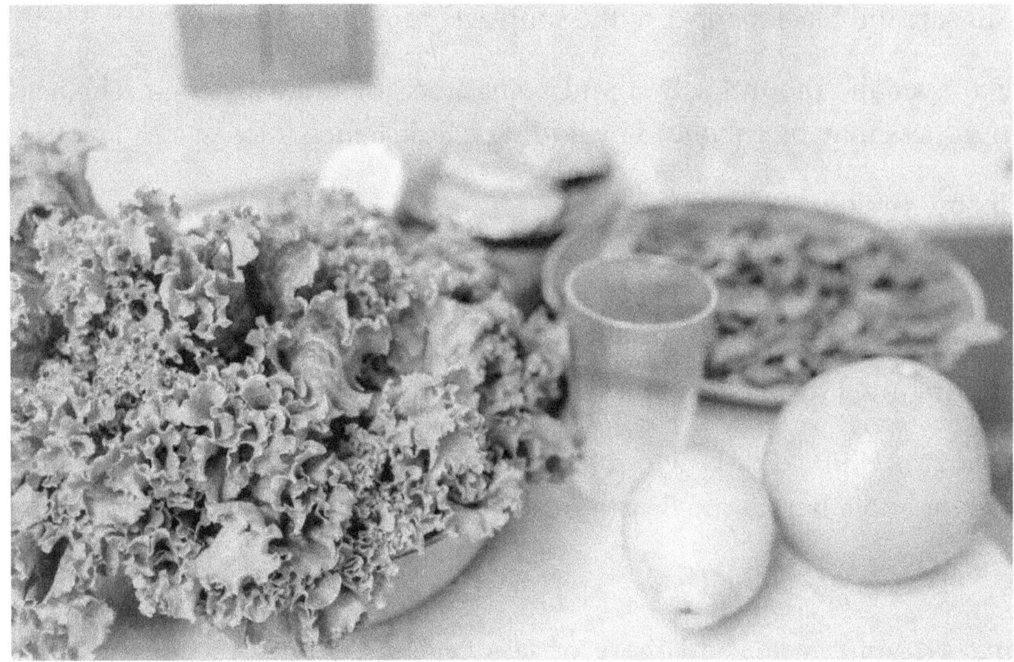

**Ingredients:**

**To make the coleslaw:**

- 4 cups of finely sliced or shredded green cabbage

- Lacinato kale (Dinosaur kale): 2 cups, cut leaves with stems removed.

- Two medium-sized shredded or julienned carrots

- Cut one small red onion into thin slices.

- For garnishing purposes, 1/4 cup of fresh parsley, chopped or unchopped.

- 1/4 cup of almonds that have been sliced (optional for an added crunch)

- To add a touch of sweetness, you may add 1/4 cup. plump cranberries

**To be Dressed:**

- **Greek yogurt:** 1/2 cup (for a vegan option, use mayonnaise or a dairy-free spread).

- **Mustard de Dijon:** 2 teaspoons

- **Vinegar of apple:** 2 teaspoons

- **Honey:** 2 tablespoons (or, for a vegan alternative, maple syrup)

- 1/2 teaspoon of salt, or more if you like it.

- For a little additional heat, add 1/4 teaspoon of black pepper.

**Instructions:**

*To make the coleslaw:*

Begin by grinding or julienning the carrots, cutting the lacinato kale after taking off the tough stems, and slicing the red onion very thinly. In a big bowl, you should mix all of these items together.

*Optional Ingredients:* Top the bowl with the slivered almonds and dried cranberries. These give the coleslaw a lovely crunch and sweetness.

**To be Dressed:**

Mix Dijon mustard, apple cider vinegar, honey (or maple syrup), salt, and black pepper in a separate bowl. This is the designated area for preparing the dressing. Make sure the sauce is well-combined and silky.

Pour the dressing over the chopped vegetables in the mixing basin to combine the cole slaw and dressing.

*Mix and Coat:* Gently mix the ingredients for the slaw with the dressing until well-coated. Make sure the dressing gets into every crevice of the kale and cabbage.

Reserve half an hour before serving by covering and chilling the coleslaw. As the cabbage and kale cook, their flavours can mellow and combine.

To add a splash of color and freshness, sprinkle the coleslaw with finely chopped fresh parsley before serving.

**Cooking Notes:**

You may alter this coleslaw to your flavor. Consider using some thinly sliced apples, red cabbage for additional color, or a scattering of sunflower seeds for texture.

Use dairy-free yogurt or mayonnaise in the dressing, and use maple syrup instead of honey to make this coleslaw vegan.

By changing the amounts of honey and apple cider vinegar, you can customize the sweetness and acidity of the dressing to suit your tastes.

Making coleslaw in advance and storing it in the fridge for a day or two is possible. It's a fantastic recipe to cook in advance for weekday dinners or picnics and barbecues.

Cabbage and kale coleslaw is a colorful and wholesome dish that puts a new spin on traditional coleslaw. The mix of green cabbage, lacinato kale, and a tangy, creamy dressing produces a balance of tastes and textures. This coleslaw adds a splash of color, crunch, and a tinge of sweetness to any menu, whether served as a side dish or a light entrée. As you appreciate each meal, please enjoy its adaptability and health advantages.

**Chapter 5: Main Dishes - Poultry and Seafood**

- **Recipe 16: Lemon and dill salmon baked in the oven**

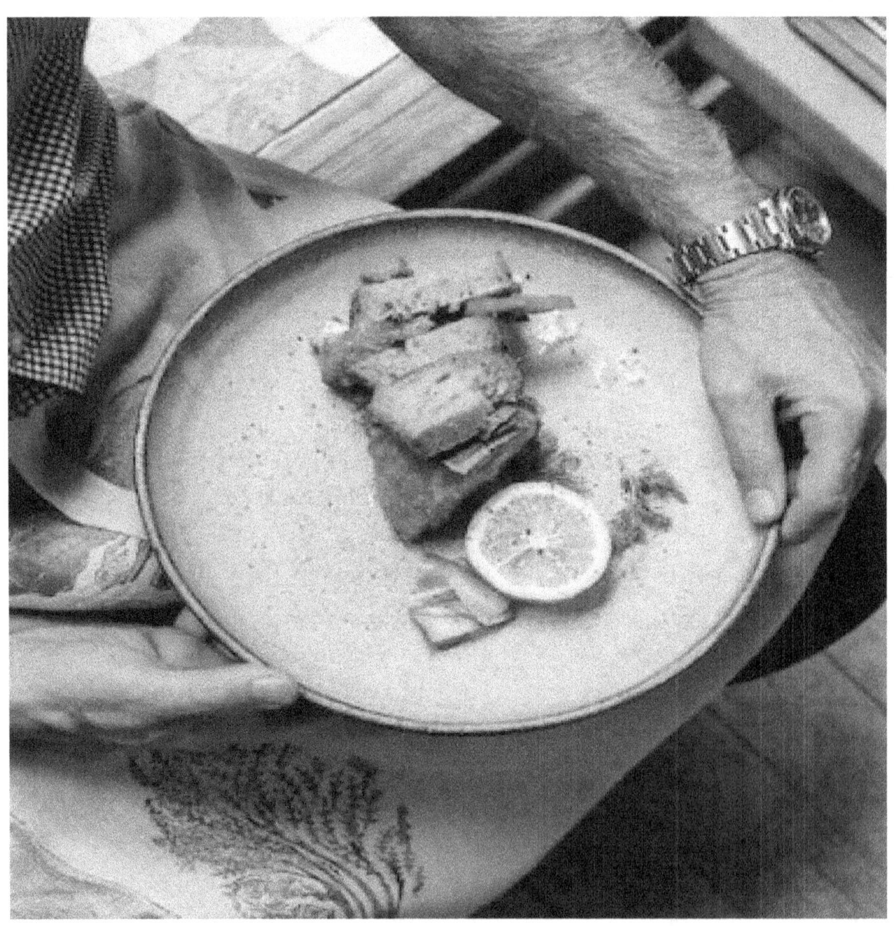

**Ingredients:**

- Salmon Filets: 4 salmon filets, each 6 to 8 ounces and with or without skin.

- Cut a big, fresh lemon into squares very carefully.

- Chopped fresh dill, 1/4 cup

- Oil from extra-virgin olives: Include 2 tablespoons

- Three or two cloves of garlic, please, chopped.

- Add salt to taste, measuring one teaspoon or more if desired.

- Add half a teaspoon of black pepper or more to taste.

**Paprika:** 1/2 teaspoon (optional, for a smokey taste)

- Adding 1/4 teaspoon of red pepper flakes may make it somewhat spicier.

- Zest of Lemon: If you want a stronger lemon taste, add the zest of one lemon.

- Lemon juice from scratch: About two to three teaspoons of lemon juice

**Instructions:**

Approximately 190 degrees Celsius (375 degrees Fahrenheit) is ideal for preheating the oven. In the middle of the oven, place a wire rack.

**Cooking filet mignon:** Drain the fish by patting it dry with paper towels. Both skinless and skinless salmon may be baked.

Add salt, pepper, and paprika to the salmon on both sides. These seasonings will bring out the best in the fish.

In a small bowl, arrange the minced dill. You may add some red pepper flakes, lemon juice, zest, and extra-virgin olive oil if you want. Mix everything. To make a fragrant and tasty mixture, stir all ingredients until they are well mixed.

**Lay out the lemon wedges:** After halving the lemon slices, lay them flat on a baking sheet covered with foil or parchment paper to make cleaning a breeze. After this, the salmon will slumber.

Season the salmon fillets and lay them on the lemon slices to create a bed of lemons. In addition to adding a tangy taste, it prevents the salmon from adhering to the baking pan.

Evenly distribute the dill and garlic mixture over the salmon fillets. Ensure that every filet is adequately coated.

Place remaining lemon slices on top of salmon filets: Dot the salmon filets with the remaining lemon slices. This enhances the look and gives the fish a more delicious lemon flavor.

*Bake:* For 15 to 20 minutes, bake the sheet in a hot oven. The exact baking time will depend on how thick your salmon filets are. When the 145°F (63°C) internal temperature is reached and the salmon easily flakes with a fork, it is done.

When serving, keep the lemon slices on top of the salmon filets after they have been cooked. Any dill and garlic mixture still on the baking sheet should be spooned over the fish.

For a beautiful display, garnish the baked salmon with more fresh dill and a few slices of lemon.

*Enjoy:* While the salmon is still warm, serve it immediately with lemon and dill. It goes well with rice, roasted vegetables, or a crisp salad as a side dish.

**Cooking Notes:**

- If you want to add more flavor and color to this dish, you may add more herbs like thyme or rosemary and sliced onions or cherry tomatoes.

- Salmon is flavored with lemon slices, which helps keep the fish wet during baking. They may be consumed with the fish to provide a zesty burst of brightness.

- Salmon may dry out if roasted for too long, but it must be regularly watched to prevent overcooking.

The traditional and delicious meal of baked salmon with lemon and dill brings out the inherent tastes of the fish while infusing it with the zesty, fresh scent of lemon and the savory flavor of dill. This recipe yields a restaurant-quality meal that is simple to make and ideal for weekday dinners or special occasions. Enjoy the succulent, flaky salmon, flavored with a delectable blend of citrus and herbs and served with vivid lemon slices for a blast of flavor with each mouthful.

- **Recipe 17: Grilled Chicken with Herbs**

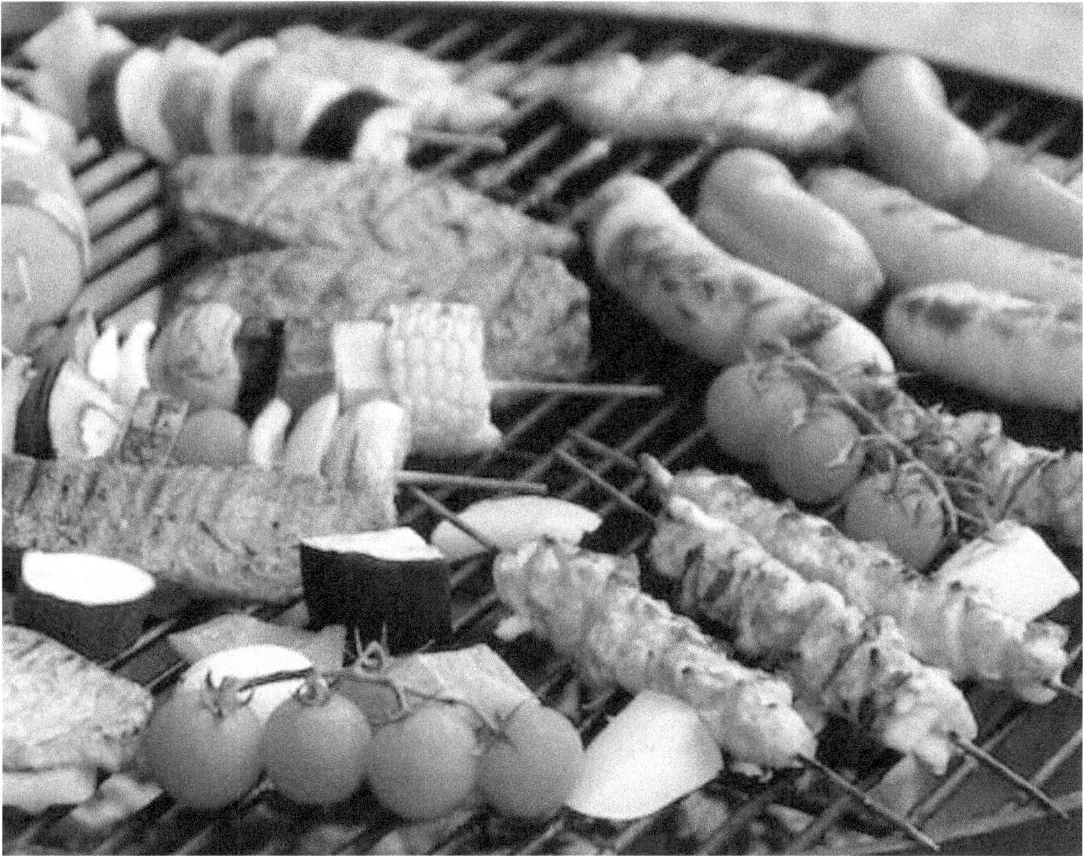

**Ingredients:**

It has four chicken breasts that are boneless and skinless. Each one weighs about 6 to 8 ounces.

- New Herbs: 1/4 cup of fresh herbs, chopped very small, like parsley, rosemary, thyme, oregano, and thyme

- Three to four garlic cloves cut up

- Zest of Lemon: One lemon's zest

- Lemon Juice: About two to three drops of lemon juice

- Oil from extra-virgin olives: half a cup

- Add salt to taste, measuring one teaspoon or more if desired.

- Add half a teaspoon of black pepper, or more to taste.

- It may be made somewhat spicier by adding 1/4 teaspoon of red pepper flakes.

**Instructions:**

Mince the garlic, chop the fresh herbs, add the zest of the lemon, and (if using) red pepper flakes. In a bowl, combine all of the marinade ingredients. Not only will this flavorful mixture season the chicken, but it may also be served as a dip.

Put the chicken breasts in a large plastic bag or a level surface to soak for a little. Pour the sauce over the chicken so it coats it completely. Place the container in the refrigerator for at least 30 minutes to allow the flavours to meld while covered or partially covered. The chicken will have an even more flavorful flavour after marinating for at least three hours or overnight.

*How to Prepare the Grill:* Adjust the grill's heat to medium-high. Grates that are clean and gently greased will not stick.

**Grill the chicken:**

1. Remove it from the sauce and let any extra run off.

2. Put the chicken breasts on the hot grill.

3. It depends on how thick the chicken is, but grill each side for 6 to 8 minutes, or until the chicken hits 165°F (74°C) and the middle is no longer pink.

4. While grilling the chicken, baste it with the leftover marinade for more flavor and moisture.

*Rest the Chicken:* Once cooked, remove the grill and set aside to rest for a few minutes. This allows for the displacement of fluids, which results in a finished product that is both juicy and tender.

*Slice and Serve:* CCut the cooked chicken breasts into long, thin pieces. To serve, put them on a dish and sprinkle with any sauce that's still left over. For extra taste and color, add more fresh herbs on top.

*Enjoy:* While it's still warm, immediately serve your grilled chicken with herbs. It goes well with grilled veggies on the side, a crisp salad, or a meal of light grains.

**Cooking Notes:**

For this recipe, you may use bone-in, skin-on chicken thighs or breasts; adjust the grilling time.

Depending on your preferences, try out various herb combinations. Use fresh basil, mint, and parsley for a Mediterranean flavor.

Soak wooden skewers in water for around half an hour before grilling to prevent burning.

Test the doneness of the chicken by inserting a meat thermometer into the thickest portion of the breast. The inside temperature should be a minimum of 165°F or 74°C.

The freshness and perfume of herbaceous marinade are infused into the chicken as it is grilled to enhance the natural taste of the chicken. Grilled chicken with herbs is a simple but exquisite recipe. This dish provides a pleasing blend of tangy lemon, fragrant herbs, and a hint of spice for a filling lunch. Whether served for a nice dinner or a casual BBQ, this grilled chicken will satisfy the audience since it delivers a flavorful explosion with each mouthful. Enjoy this meal of grilled chicken, which is juicy, tender, and flavored with herbs.

- **Recipe 18: Shrimp and Vegetable Stir-Fry**

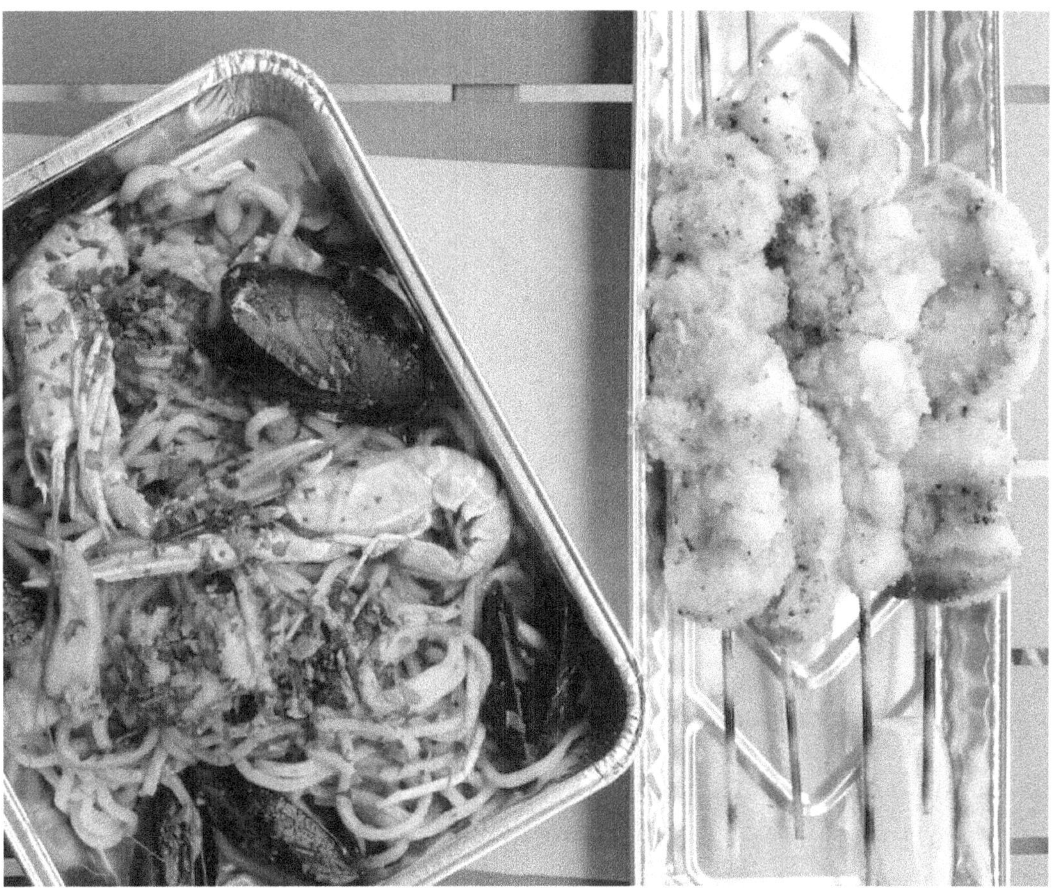

**Ingredients:**

*When making the stir-fry sauce:*

- A quarter cup of soy sauce

- One tablespoon of maple syrup (or two teaspoons of honey for vegans)

- Vinegar of rice: two teaspoons

- One tablespoon of sesame oil

- Two tablespoons of cornstarch

- 1 inch piece of grated fresh ginger

- Three to four minced cloves of garlic

- 1 and a half teaspoons of red pepper flakes (add more or less according to your preference)

**The stir-fry:**

- 1 pound of big shrimp that have been peeled and gutted

- 4 cups of mixed veggies, sliced or chopped (bell peppers, broccoli, snap peas, carrots, and any other vegetables you like).

- Dozens of drops of food oil, like peanut or veggie oil

- To taste, add 1/2 teaspoon of salt.

- For a little additional heat, add 1/4 teaspoon of black pepper.

- Sesame Seeds: An optional garnish

- Chopped green onions as a garnish (optional)

- *Rice or noodles that have been cooked:*

**Instructions:**

*When making the stir-fry sauce:*

Gather the ingredients in a small bowl and combine the rice vinegar, soy sauce, honey (or maple syrup), cornstarch, minced garlic, sesame oil, the fresh ginger that was handed to you, and red pepper flakes. You may customize the heat level to your preference. Your stir-fry sauce will be delicious thanks to this mixture.

*The stir-fry:*

*Shrimp preparation:* Thaw frozen shrimp in a strainer and pour cold water over it. With paper towels, dry the shrimp. Black pepper and a dash of salt are used to season the shrimp.

Add the oil to the pan and set it over medium-high heat to begin heating. To make the oil shimmer, stir it around.

*Sear the Shrimp:* In the hot pan, spread the shrimp that has been seasoned out in a single layer. For about one to two minutes on each side, until thick and pink. Take the cooked shrimp out of the pan and set it away.

*Vegetable Stir-Fry:* If you need to, add oil to the same pan before adding the chopped or sliced vegetables. Stir-fry them for about five to seven minutes, or until they are crisp-tender and beginning to turn brown.

Return the shrimp to the stir-fried vegetable mixture and toss with the sauce once cooked. Add the prepared stir-fry sauce and mix well. Tossing the ingredients together will ensure that the sauce is distributed evenly.

*Cooking to Thicken:* For two to three minutes, or until it gets thick and shiny, cook the sauce. Stir it all the time so it doesn't stick.

When the sauce has reached the desired consistency and the shrimp and veggies are covered, remove the skillet from the heat to serve.

Top your stir-fried shrimp and vegetables with sesame seeds and finely chopped green onions if preferred. These provide a delicious crunch and flavorful freshness.

Your shrimp and vegetable stir-fry should be served with hot, over-cooked rice or noodles. The sauce will provide savory and faintly sweet tastes to the grains.

**Cooking Notes:**

Please put your favorite veggies in your stir-fry to make it your own. You may mix other vegetables that you want, such as colorful bell peppers, broccoli florets, snap peas, carrots, and mushrooms.

Use gluten-free tamari or soy sauce to convert this dish to a gluten-free diet.

Use other ingredients like cashews, sliced almonds, or water chestnuts for more texture and taste.

By adjusting the quantity of red pepper flakes or using a chili oil dab, you may alter the degree of heat.

Shrimp and veggie stir-fried in a pan can be a main dish or a side dish for other Asian-style meals.

The shrimp and vegetable stir-fry is a quick, tasty, and healthy recipe. It has tiny shrimp, a variety of brightly colored fresh vegetables, and a savory and slightly sweet stir-fry sauce on top. The harmonious blend of textures and tastes in this recipe makes it ideal for a satisfying midweek supper or for a fast and simple meal whenever you need one. Enjoy the different tastes and the freedom to make it your own.

- **Recipe 19: Lemon Herb Turkey Breast**

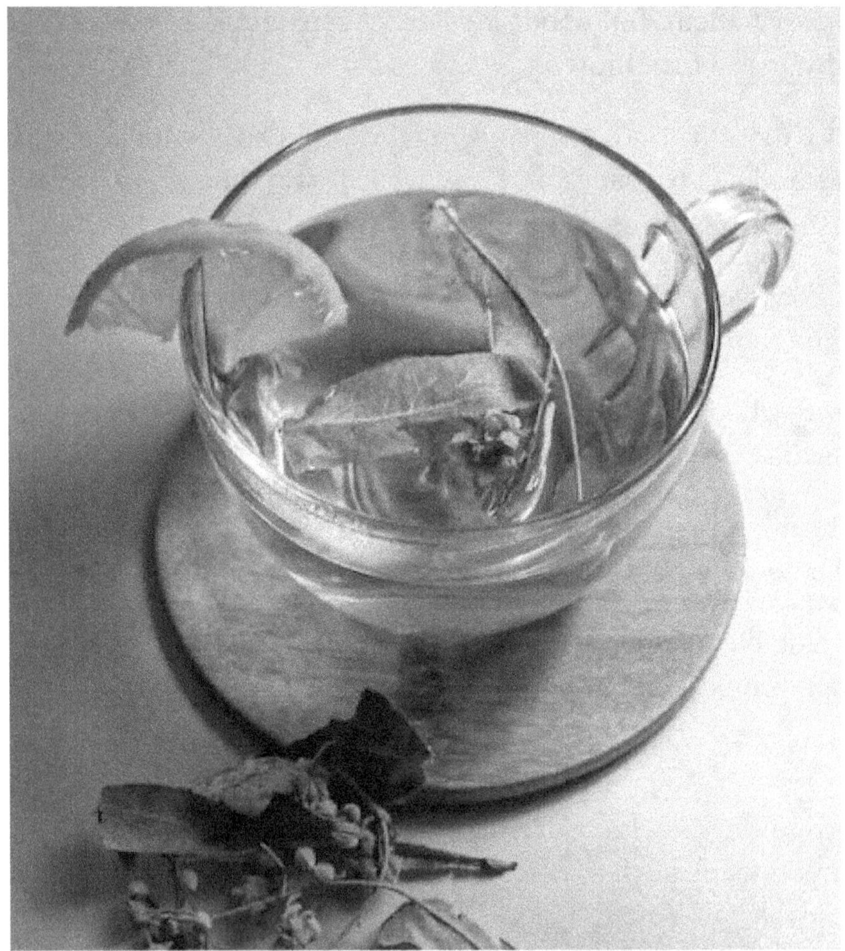

**Ingredients:**

- For the marinade for the turkey:

- One boneless turkey breast (about 2-3 pounds)

- Fresh lemon: one lemon's zest

- Fresh lemon juice: About 2-3 teaspoons of juice from one lemon

- Ground or chopped 1/4 cup of fresh herbs (such as rosemary, parsley, thyme, oregano, or parsley) will go into the sauce.

- Three to four garlic cloves cut up

- Measure 1/4 cup of extra virgin olive oil.

- Add salt to taste, measuring one teaspoon or more if desired.

- 1/2 teaspoon of black pepper, or more if you like

**When roasting:**

Fresh lemon slices: one lemon

*Fresh Herbs:* A few sprigs of fresh herbs of your choosing, such as rosemary or thyme

*Basting liquid:* half a cup of chicken or turkey broth

Wrap the turkey breast with cooking thread for a secure hold.

**Instructions:**

*For the marinade for the turkey:*

Blend fresh lemon juice, zest, minced garlic, chopped herbs, extra-virgin olive oil, salt, and black pepper in a bowl. You may marinate turkey breast in this delicious mixture or use it as a dipping sauce.

*The Turkey:*

Wash the turkey breast under cold water and dry it well with paper towels before cooking. As long as the skin isn't too thick, you may roast turkey breasts with the skin on.

Prepare the turkey breast in a small dish or a large zip-top bag. Pour the sauce over the turkey, covering the breast completely. Refrigerate for at least two hours, preferably overnight, after sealing the bag or covering the dish. It will aid in the blending of flavours.

*Warm up.* The oven should be heated up to 325 degrees Fahrenheit (163 degrees Celsius). In the center of the oven, position a rack.

*Bind the Turkey (Optional):* To help the turkey roast evenly, if the thickness of the breast is uneven, bind it with cooking twine. At 1-inch intervals, tie the string around the bird.

*Roast Turkey:* Sprinkle a baking dish or skillet with fresh lemon slices and herb leaves as a foundation. If the turkey breast has any skin, place it skin-side up on top.

To spread and cook, add the chicken or turkey stock to the pan. This will keep the turkey breast moist while it's cooking. Once the turkey breast hits 165°F (74°C) on the inside and the skin is golden brown and crisp, put the pan in a hot oven and roast for one to one and a half hours. Brush the turkey breast with the pan juices every 30 minutes to make it taste better and stay moist.

The turkey should be removed from the oven and allowed to rest for about 15 minutes before slicing once it has cooked through. While the liquids are being moved around, the turkey breast stays fresh and tasty. After taking out any string, cut the turkey into thin slices.

Place the sliced lemon-herb turkey breast on a serving tray, garnish with more fresh herbs, and serve immediately. It goes well with preferred sides, such as mashed potatoes, roasted veggies, or a crisp salad.

**Cooking Notes:**

Adapt the herbs to your preferences. You may utilize a single herb type or a mix of herbs based on your preferences.

To make gravy, deglaze the roasting pan with white wine or turkey stock and thicken it with a cornstarch slurry.

Use a meat thermometer while roasting a turkey to check the internal temperature and prevent overcooking, which may lead to dry flesh.

Leftover lemon-herb turkey breast is excellent for adding protein to salads, sandwiches, and wraps.

A delicious and flavorful meal, lemon herb turkey breast brings out the inherent turkey characteristics while infusing them with the zesty, herbaceous flavor of lemon and fresh herbs. This dinner is a treat for every occasion, not just a show-stopper for holiday feasts. This roasted turkey breast is delicious and goes well with your favorite sides. It is soft, juicy, and flavored with herbs.

- **Recipe 20: Quinoa-Crusted Tilapia**

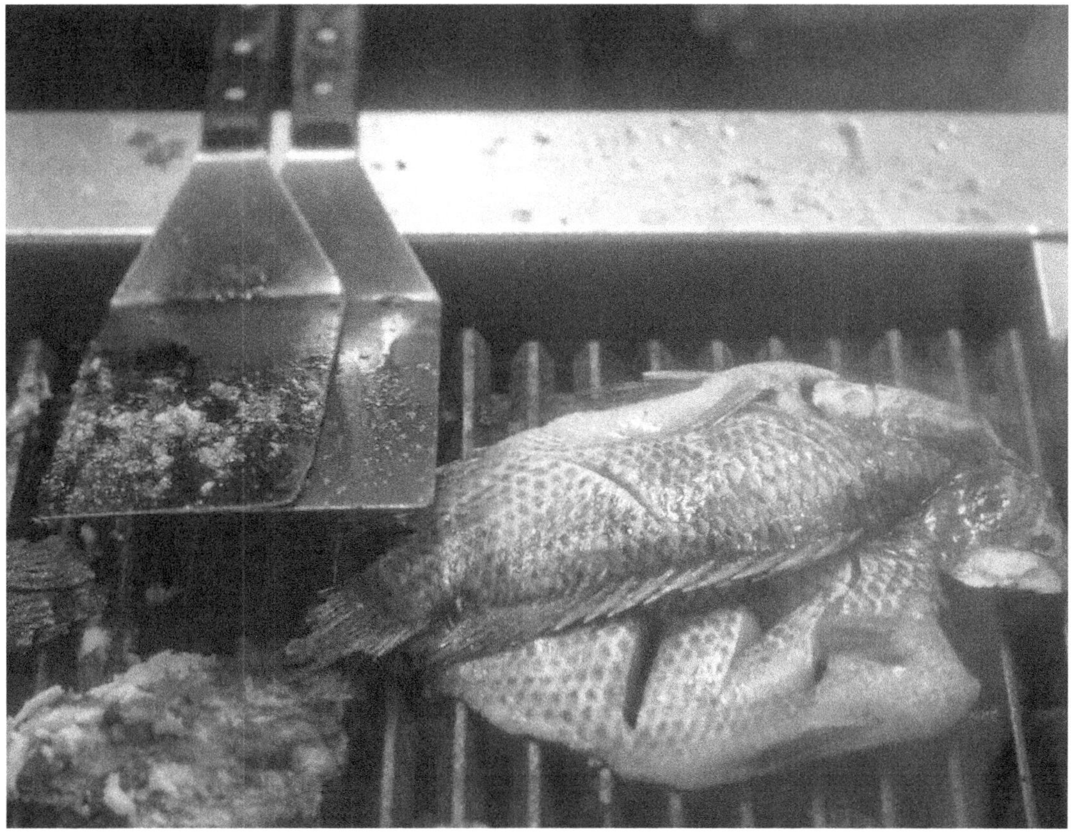

**Ingredients:**

- With regard to the quinoa crust:

- 100 milliliters of fast-cooked rice

- Panko breadcrumbs, 1/2 cup

- 1/4 cup of finely grated Parmesan

- Minced fresh herbs, about two teaspoons worth. Fresh herbs like parsley, cilantro, or basil will do.

- Powdered garlic: 1/2 teaspoon

- fifty-two milliliters of salt

- one-fourth teaspoon of black pepper

- Distilled olive oil, two millilitres

**The tilapia:**

- The weight of the four tilapia filets is around 6 to 8 ounces.

- 1.5 cups of all-purpose flour

- One large beaten egg (1 egg)

- 

- Two teaspoons of oil for frying in a pan

- Zesty lemon slices, for presentation purposes only

- Garnish with fresh herbs if desired

**Instructions:**

*Regarding the quinoa crust:*

Before cooking quinoa, rinse it well under cold running water. The quinoa and two cups of water are combined in a medium-sized saucepan. Bring the mixture to a boil after the quinoa has finished cooking and absorbed all the water. Next, reduce the heat to low, cover the pan, and cook for 15 to 20 minutes. Before letting the cooked quinoa cool, give it a little fluff with a fork?

Coarsely chop some fresh herbs and add them to a large bowl with the cooked quinoa, panko breadcrumbs, sliced Parmesan cheese, salt, and black pepper to form the crust. After adding the olive oil, mix all ingredients well. A little bit of water should be added to the mixture.

*The tilapia:*

How to prepare tilapia filets: Dry the fish filets with paper towels. On both sides of each filet, sprinkle a little salt and black pepper.

Coat in a shallow dish that has been dusted with all-purpose flour. Once dredged in the flour, coat each tilapia filet equally. Get rid of any excess flour.

Tilapia filets that have been breaded should be dipped into a beaten egg, letting any excess fall off.

Apply Quinoa Crust: Press each tilapia filet with an egg coating into the quinoa crust mixture, making sure the crust sticks to the fish on all sides. To get a consistent crust, gently apply the quinoa mixture to the filets.

**Pan-Fry:**

1.  Melt the oil in a large skillet over medium-high heat.

2.  Carefully add the quinoa-coated fish filets to the heated oil.

Once the crust becomes golden and the fish reaches the desired doneness, fry the tilapia on each side for three to four minutes. When the fish reaches an internal temperature of 145°F (63°C) and readily flakes when tested with a fork, it is considered done.


Before you garnish and serve the tilapia filets with quinoa crust, take them out of the pan and set them on a serving platter. Slices of lemon and fresh herbs may be used as garnishes if desired.

*Enjoy:* While the tilapia with quinoa crust is still hot and crispy, serve it immediately. A side of steamed veggies, a crisp salad, or a zesty sauce goes well with it.

**Cooking Notes:**

Feel free to experiment with various herbs and flavors for the quinoa crust. You may also mix in a little paprika, cayenne, or lemon zest for added taste.

Before adding the tilapia filets to the pan, ensure the frying oil is hot. This aids in producing a crispy crust.

Fish with a quinoa crust is a healthy alternative; bake it for 15–20 minutes or until done and brown on top. Get the oven up to 400 degrees Fahrenheit (200 degrees Celsius).

Quinoa-crusted tilapia is a tasty and healthy meal that combines the mild and crispy texture of tilapia with the crunchy, nutty texture of quinoa. This dish is a versatile choice for a healthy meal because it blends tastes and textures so well. Enjoy the delicate fish filets and the crunchy crust that is flavored with herbs. They make a tasty and healthy dinner.

- **Recipe 21: Chickpea and Spinach Curry**

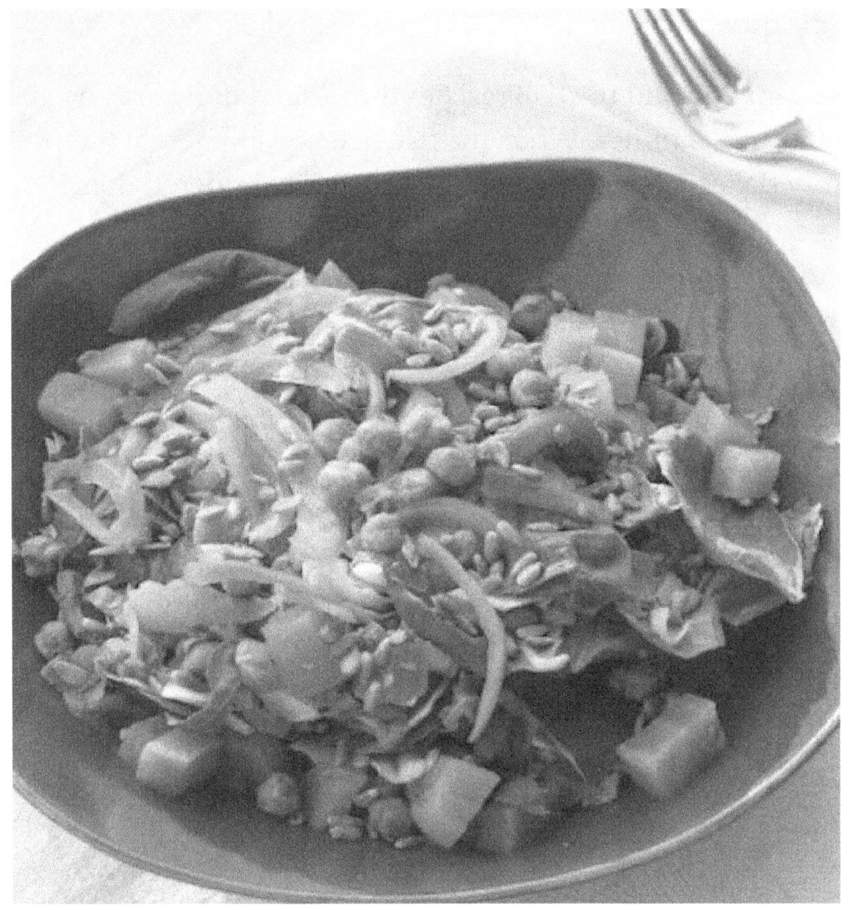

**Ingredients:**

- Two 15-ounce cans of chickpeas, cleaned and drained, or three cups of cooked chickpeas.

- 6 cups of fresh spinach pieces that are cut up pretty big

- One large onion, cut up very small

- 3 to 4 garlic cloves, chopped up

- 1 inch chunk of chopped ginger

- For two medium-sized tomatoes, chop them up. You can also use canned diced tomatoes.

- Can of coconut milk, 13.5 oz.

- Two tablespoons of cooking oil, like veggie or coconut oil

- Add or take away two teaspoons of curry powder.

- Half a teaspoon of turmeric powder

- One teaspoon of cumin seeds

- Ground coriander, measuring half a teaspoon

- According to your preference, add or remove 1/4 teaspoon of chile pepper.

- Add salt to taste, measuring one teaspoon or more if desired.

- 1/2 teaspoon of black pepper, or more if you like

- Use fresh cilantro as a garnish

- Naan bread or cooked rice: Both are brought out.

**Instructions:**

Heat the oil in a large saucepan over medium-low heat. Sauté the aromatics. Chop the onion finely and throw it in the pan. After around 5 minutes of sautéing, the onion should become somewhat brown and translucent.

Stir in the garlic and ginger that have been grated. Add a minute or two of sautéing time to make sure the food starts to smell delicious.

Take it to the next level by seasoning the simmering aromas with ground cumin, coriander, turmeric, ground cumin, ground chilli pepper (if using), salt, and black pepper. A plethora of spices should be blended with the ginger, garlic, and onions. Toasting the spices for a minute or two is all it takes to bring out their flavour.

Chopped tomatoes (or canned diced tomatoes) should be added to the pan. Allow the tomatoes to soften and release their juices for 5 to 7 minutes, creating a fragrant and flavorful tomato foundation.

Simmering Coconut Milk:

1. Incorporate the can of coconut milk by whisking it.

2. Place the mixture over low heat and bring to a simmer.

3. Simmer for 5 to 7 minutes to let the flavours combine, and the sauce thicken.

After the chickpeas have been drained and rinsed, add them to the pan. After adding them to the sauce and simmering for 5 to 7 minutes, they should be cooked thoroughly and seasoned with curry.

Add some spinach by slowly mixing in the chopped fresh or frozen spinach, depending on your preference. The spinach needs around three to five minutes to wilt and cook through.

Add more salt, black pepper, or cayenne to taste after tasting the curry. Adjust seasonings to suit personal preference.

Dish out the chickpea and spinach stew and serve. For a vibrant and stimulating garnish, try using fresh cilantro leaves.

**Serve with Hot Rice or Naan:** This chickpea and spinach curry goes well with hot rice and warm naan bread for a hearty and satisfying supper.

**Cooking Notes:**

Change the quantity of cayenne pepper in the curry to suit your preferred degree of heat. If you want a milder curry, leave it out entirely.

Add more veggies like bell peppers, peas, or carrots for more nutrition and diversity.

Use vegetable oil and confirm that your canned coconut milk is devoid of any substances originating from animals to make this meal vegan.

The following day's lunch may be made from leftovers chilled for a day or two.

The earthy richness of chickpeas and the vivid green deliciousness of spinach are combined in a tasty and filling curry sauce to create chickpea and spinach curry. In addition to being vegetarian and filling, this dish is quick and simple to make. This curry's hearty warmth and bold flavors make for a delightful supper that can be enjoyed any day of the week. It goes well with rice or naan.

- **Recipe 22: Stuffed Bell Peppers with Quinoa and Black Beans**

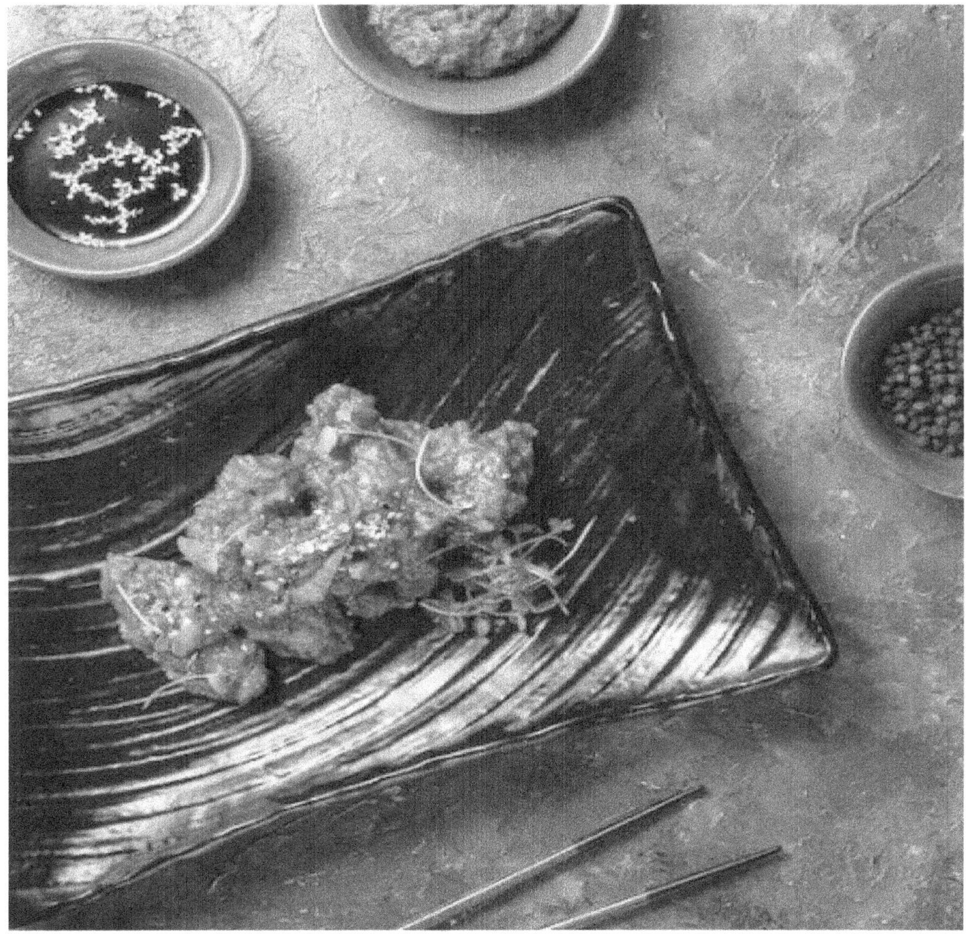

Ingredients:

- **Concerning the filled peppers:**

- **Red peppers:** 4. Four large bell peppers, any shade

- 100 milliliters of fast-cooked rice

- **Cooked black beans:** 1 can (15 ounces) or 1.5 cups (after draining and rinsing).

- Corn kernels, fresh, frozen, or canned, measuring 1 cup

- A medium-sized onion, roughly chopped

- minced garlic cloves (three or four)

- Half a grape's worth of tomatoes

- A teaspoon of seasoning

- Swipe the one teaspoon of chilli powder to add or remove.

- To taste, add 1/2 teaspoon of salt.

- Add more black pepper to taste, up to 1/4 teaspoon. more heat

- Distilled olive oil, two millilitres

- A quarter cup of fresh parsley, roughly chopped

- If desired, garnish with 1/2 cup of shredded cheese.

- Concerning the sauce made from tomatoes:

- Thirteen fluid ounces of tomato sauce is in one can.

- Chopped garlic, one or two cloves

- Dried oregano, one teaspoonful.

- To taste, add 1/2 teaspoon of salt.

- Add more black pepper to taste, up to 1/4 teaspoon. more heat

**Instructions:**

To prepare the quinoa for the Stuffed Peppers, give it a good rinse under cold running water. The quinoa and two cups of water are combined in a medium-sized saucepan. Bring the mixture to a boil after the quinoa has finished cooking and absorbed all the water. Next, reduce the heat to low, cover the pan, and cook for 15 to 20 minutes. Before letting the cooked quinoa cool, give it a little fluff with a fork?

**Get ready.** Get the oven to a hot temperature, around 190 degrees Celsius (375 degrees Fahrenheit). In the centre of the oven, position a rack.

**Cut off the tops and scoop :**

1. Cut the membranes and seeds to prepare the bell peppers.

2. Cut the peppers' bottoms if required so they can stand straight in a baking dish.

Season the peppers with a little olive oil and set them aside.

**Sauté the Aromatics:**

1. Two tablespoons of olive oil, heated over medium heat in a big skillet or saucepan.

2. Chop the onion finely and throw it in the pan. For a little browning and a transparent onion, sauté for around 5 minutes.

3. When the garlic smells wonderful, add the chopped garlic and stir for one or two more minutes.

**Tomatoes and seasonings:** Toss the diced tomatoes and seasonings in the pan. To get the tomatoes soft, simmer for around 5–7 minutes. Cumin, chilli powder, salt, and black pepper should be added afterwards. Thoroughly blend.

Combine the cooked rice, black beans (after rinsing and draining), corn kernels, and tomato sauce (from the pan) in a large bowl. Add the quinoa and stir well. Ensure that the ingredients are well-mixed.

**Stuff the Bell Peppers:** Carefully pour the rice and black bean mixture into each pepper, pushing down to fill. You could worry about placing too much in each pepper since the middle tends to settle when baking.

Combine the canned tomato sauce with the minced garlic, dry oregano, salt, and black pepper in another bowl. Here is the recipe for tomato sauce. To prepare the sauce, combine all of the ingredients well.

After placing the stuffed bell peppers on a baking tray, please stand up and bake them. Pour the tomato sauce over the peppers until they are completely coated. Cover the baking dish with aluminium foil.

Remove the dish after 30–35 minutes of baking in the oven. After 10–15 minutes of baking without the paper, the peppers should be tender and the tops lightly browned.

If using, for 5 minutes in the oven, top each stuffed bell pepper with shredded cheese. This step is entirely optional. Allow the cheese to melt and bubble for a little.

The stuffed bell peppers are ready to be served once taken out of the oven and adorned. Garnish with chopped cilantro that is just picked up.

Please take pleasure in: Before topping off your quinoa and black bean-filled bell peppers with more tomato sauce, warm them up.

**Cooking Notes:**

Add other veggies, such as sliced zucchini, mushrooms, or chopped spinach, to the filling to suit your tastes.

You may top the dish with the cheese of your choice, such as cheddar, Monterey Jack, or a dairy-free substitute if you're a vegan.

You can put the extras in the fridge for one or two days and eat them for lunch the next day.

A substantial, tasty dish that blends the sweetness of bell peppers with a protein-rich filling is stuffed bell peppers with quinoa and black beans. This dish is a wonderful option for a healthy supper or meal preparation since it delivers a nice combination of textures and flavors. This meal will warm your heart and satisfy your hunger as you take in its brilliant colors and strong tastes.

- **Recipe 23: Portobello Mushroom Burgers**

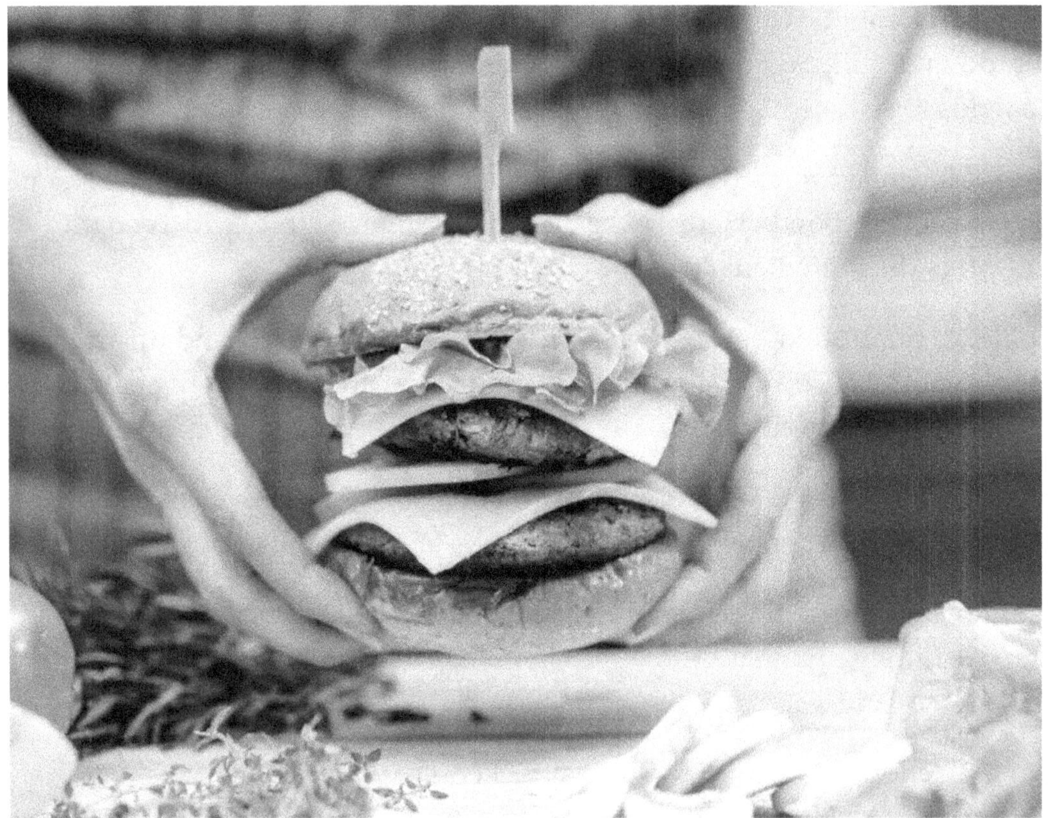

**Ingredients:**

*Used for the Marina de Portobello:*

- Four large, clean portobello mushroom caps without stems

- 1/4 cup vinegar made from grapes

- Two milliliters of olive oil

- Two tablespoons of soy sauce (or tamari if you can't have gluten)

- Please chop two to three garlic cloves.

- One teaspoon of dried oregano.

- Half a teaspoon of kosher salt

- Salt to taste, 1/4 teaspoon or more.

- The Burger Assembly What's needed:

- 4 burger buns (pick your best or a whole-grain kind).

- A few new greens or spinach leaves

- Tomato slices: 1 to 2 tomatoes cut very thinly

- Red onion slices: 1 small red onion, cut into thin slices

- Two or one very thinly sliced avocados

- Four slices of cheese (you can pick the kind you like best).

- **Condiments:** Your choice of ketchup, mustard, mayonnaise, or other burger toppings

**Instructions:**

*Applied to the Portobello Marinade:*

Balsamic vinegar, olive oil, soy sauce (or tamari), chopped garlic, dried oregano, black pepper, and salt should be combined in a small bowl. Your portobello mushrooms will be marinated in a delicious sauce using this.

After you've cleaned the Portobello caps, please place them in a large zip-top bag or a sturdy plate. Cover the mushrooms completely with the sauce by pouring it over them. The flavours will blend better if you chill it for at least half an hour. The next step is to seal the bag or place a lid on the dish. Soaking for at least two hours will improve the flavour.

*Portobello mushrooms should be grilled or cooked as follows:*

Set the grill or a big pan on medium-high heat and begin cooking. You can use olive oil to keep things from sticking in the pan.

Place the marinated Portobello mushroom caps, gill side down, on the heated grill or skillet. The mushrooms should be grilled or cooked for approximately 4-5 minutes on each side until they are fork-tender and have grill marks. Extra marinade may be brushed on while cooking to enhance flavor.

**The Portobello Mushroom Burgers' construction:**

The burger buns should be gently browned after being grilled or toasted.

Scatter a few fresh lettuce or spinach leaves on the bottom of each toasted bun.

Add a Portobello mushroom cap to the greens.

On top of the mushrooms, place slices of tomato, avocado, and red onion (if using).

You can add a piece of any cheese you like to the mushroom caps that are already hot and let it melt a bit if you want to.

The top half of the toasted buns should be spread with your preferred condiments.

Place the top bun and condiments on top of the stacked components to assemble the burgers.

If necessary, fasten the burgers with toothpicks and serve right away.

**Cooking Notes:**

Pickles, roasted red peppers, and caramelized onions are a few more toppings you may add to your Portobello mushroom burgers to make them more unique.

With the savory Portobello mushrooms, try out different kinds of cheese to find the one you like best.

Without a grill or pan, you may roast the Portobello mushrooms in an oven preheated to 400 degrees Fahrenheit (200 degrees Celsius) for twenty to twenty-five minutes.

If you don't want to eat gluten, use gluten-free burger buns and make sure your soy sauce or tamari is also gluten-free.

Burgers made with portobello mushrooms are a tasty and filling substitute for regular beef burgers. Fresh and crisp veggies, meaty Portobello mushrooms marinated in balsamic and herbs, and your preferred burger toppings are all included in this dish.

Enjoy these mushroom burgers' robust, umami-rich taste as they provide a vegetarian twist to traditional burger food. They make a delicious complement to your next BBQ or are ideal for a vegetarian supper.

- **Recipe 24: Vegan Lentil Shepherd's Pie**

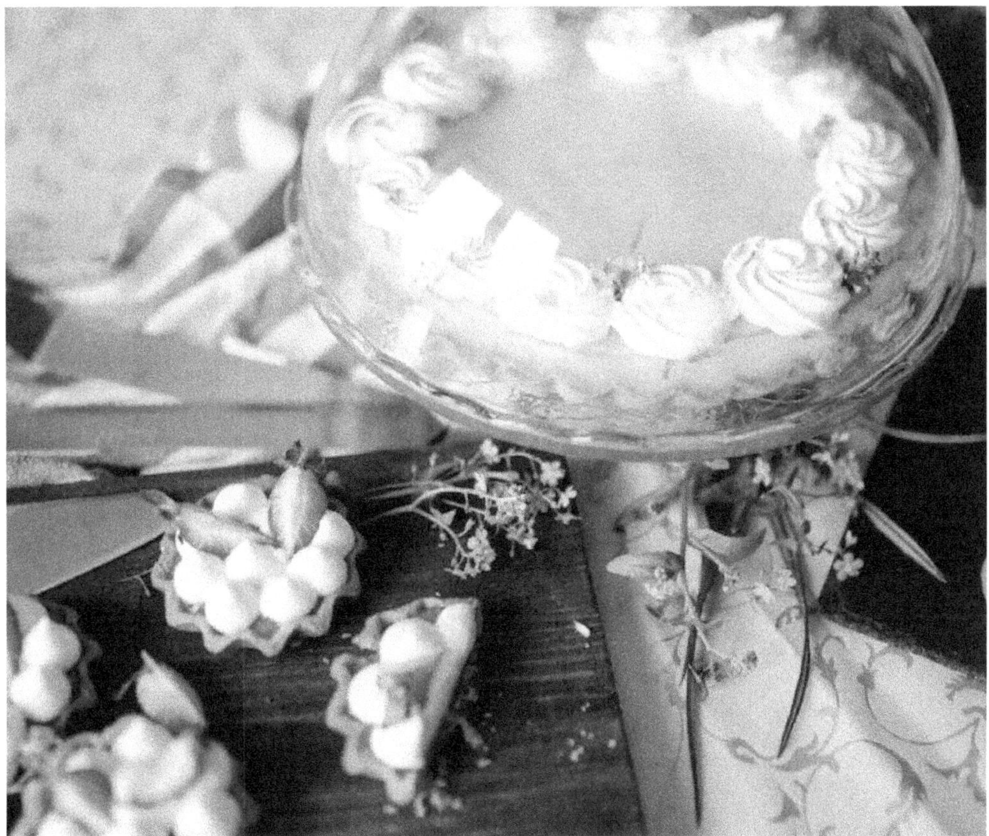

**Ingredients:**

- Regarding the lentil filling

- Green or brown lentils, 1 cup, washed and drained

- 4 cups of vegetable broth

- One big, finely chopped onion

- Two medium-sized carrots chopped

- Celery: 2 diced stalks

- Three to four minced cloves of garlic

- 1 cup frozen peas

- Two teaspoons of tomato paste

- Use either half a teaspoon of dried or one teaspoon of fresh thyme leaves.

- One or half a teaspoon of fresh or dried rosemary, depending on your preference

- One teaspoon of salt, or as much as you like

- 1/2 teaspoon of black pepper, or more if you like

- Two milliliters of olive oil

- Mashed potato topping:

- Four large potatoes, cut into cubes after being peeled

- Half a cup of almond milk that hasn't been sweetened (or any other non-dairy milk you like)

- Two to three teaspoons of vegan butter

- To taste, add 1/2 teaspoon of salt.

- For a little additional heat, add 1/4 teaspoon of black pepper.

- For a cheesy taste, you can add two tablespoons of nutritional yeast.

**Instructions:**

*Regarding the lentil filling*

If you want to cook lentils, put clean lentils and veggie soup in a big pot. Turn down the heat to a simmer after the water has boiled. For twenty to twenty-five minutes, or until soft but not mushy, cook the lentils with the lid on. After letting any extra water run off, the cooked lentils should be set away.

**Sauté Vegetables:**

1. Warm the olive oil in a big skillet over medium-low heat.

2. Incorporate the finely chopped carrots, celery, and onion.

3. After around five to seven minutes of cooking, the veggies should be tender and the onion translucent.

Add Garlic and Tomato Paste: Add the tomato paste and stir it in. Simmer for one to two minutes, or until the smell is nice. Add the tomato paste all the way through.

Season to taste, then add the cooked lentils and the vegetables that have been sautéed to the pan. Put in the black pepper, salt, rosemary, and thyme. Mix everything together completely. Simmer the mixture for two to three minutes to bring out all the flavors. If the mix seems too dry, you can add some veggie broth.

Fold the frozen peas gently and simmer for two to three minutes to fully thaw them. The lentil filling should be placed aside after turning off the stove.

**Topping made of mashed potatoes:**

Toss the diced potatoes into a big saucepan of salted water and bring to a boil. To make potatoes that can be easily pierced with a fork, soak them for at least 15 to 20 minutes.

To make mashed potatoes, drain the potatoes and then add them to the pot. Shake them up with your hand or a potato masher. Salt, black pepper, nutritional yeast (if using), and almond milk should all be added. Keep beating and mixing the potatoes until they are smooth and creamy. Change the spices to your liking.

**Build and Bake:**

Set the oven to 200 °C (400 °F).

*Filling Layers:* Spread the lentil filling out evenly in a baking dish that is 9x13 inches or a similar size.

Sprinkle the mashed potato mix over the lentil filling and use a spoon to make it round. You can use a fork to make pretty circles on top if you want to.

*Cook:* The recipe for shepherd's pie should remain unchanged. Cook it in the oven for twenty-five to thirty minutes, or until the edges are bubbling and the top is browned.

*Cool Slightly:* Allow the pie to cool down after taking it out of the oven before serving.

*Serving suggestions:* If wanted, serve your hot vegan lentil shepherd's pie with a green salad or steamed veggies.

**Cooking Notes:**

For more flavor, you may add a dash of garlic powder, chives, or other preferred herbs to the mashed potato topping.

Use whichever kind of lentils you choose, but remember to modify the cooking time since certain varieties may take longer or shorter to cook than green or brown lentils.

You can put leftovers in the fridge in a container that won't let air in for a few days and then reheat them for other meals.

The tasty and plant-based vegan lentil shepherd's pie is a warming and filling variation on the traditional meal. This recipe's combination of soft lentils, a variety of veggies, and a creamy buttery mashed potato topping produces a hearty and filling supper. Enjoy the rich, savory tastes and creamy texture as you appreciate each piece of this vegan comfort food. It's ideal for intimate family gatherings or special events.

- **Recipe 25: Sweet Potato and Black Bean Enchiladas**

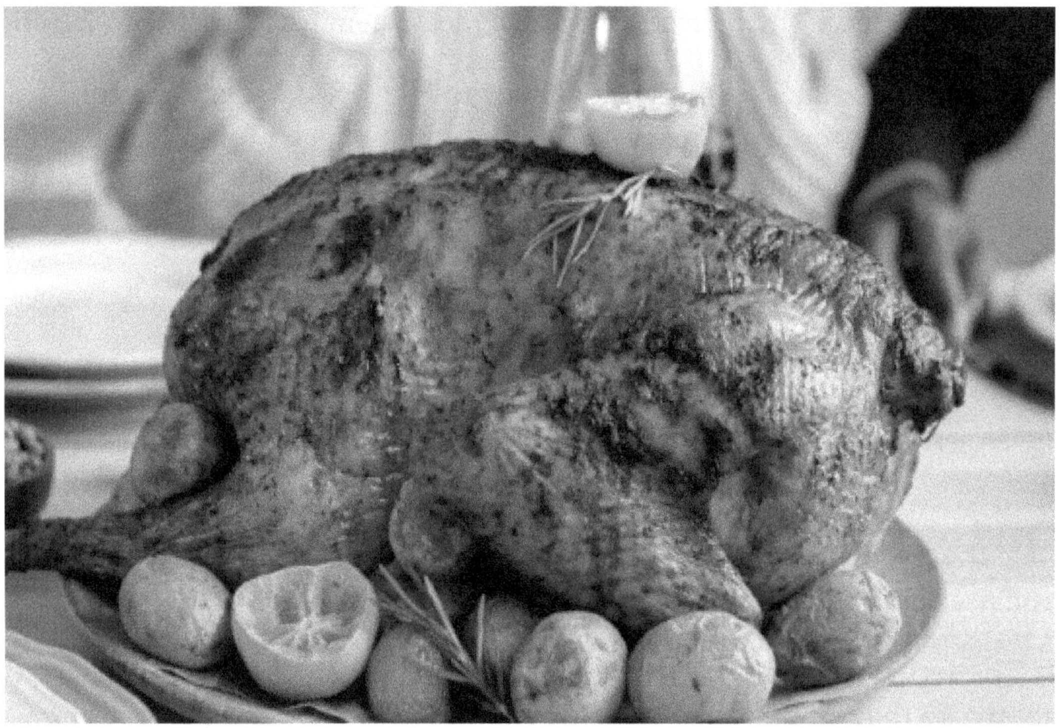

**Ingredients:**

*For the filling of the enchiladas:*

- Two golf-ball-sized sweet potatoes, peeled and diced into little chunks.

- Cooked black beans: 1 can (15 ounces) or 1.5 cups (after draining and rinsing).

- One tiny, finely sliced red onion

- Three to four minced cloves of garlic

- 2 cups chopped fresh spinach

**Cumin seed:** 1 teaspoon

- Swipe the one teaspoon of chilli powder to add or remove.

- To taste, add 1/2 teaspoon of salt.

- For a little additional heat, add 1/4 teaspoon of black pepper.

- Distilled olive oil, two millilitres

- Concerning the enchilada sauce:

- Thirteen fluid ounces of tomato sauce is in one can.

- Adjust the chilli powder proportions to your preference.

- Sumatran spice, measured in teaspoons

- Garlic powder, 1/2 teaspoon

- Add half a teaspoon of dried oregano.

- To taste, add 1/2 teaspoon of salt.

- For a little additional heat, add 1/4 teaspoon of black pepper.

- Assembling the enchiladas:

- Eight to ten corn buns, each six inches in diameter

- One cup of vegan cheese crumbles

- A quarter cup of fresh parsley, roughly chopped

- Slice some jalapenos and use them as a garnish.

- **Instructions:**

*For the filling of the enchiladas:*

Roasting sweet potatoes requires an oven temperature of 400°F or 200°C. Season the chopped sweet potatoes with salt and pepper and drizzle with olive oil. Could you put them in an ovenproof dish? Drop the outerwear. Roast the sweet potatoes in the oven for 20 to 25 minutes or until they soften and caramelize.

Heat two tablespoons of olive oil in a big pot or pan over medium heat. Add the onions and garlic and cook them until they are soft. Dice the red onion and add it. Cook for two to three minutes, or until the onion turns clear. Add the chopped garlic and stir for another minute or two, until the garlic smells good.

The spices and spinach should be added. The spinach should be cooked for two to three minutes until it wilts. Put in the salt, chili powder, cumin powder, and black pepper. Do a good mix.

Roasted sweet potatoes and black beans should be added to the pan along with the beans. Gently combine everything, then heat through for two to three minutes. Enchilada filling is removed from the heat and placed aside.

**Regarding the enchilada sauce:**

To prepare the sauce, a small saucepan should be filled with tomato sauce, chilli powder, cumin, garlic powder, salt, black pepper, dried oregano, and cumin. Swirl it constantly as it heats for around 5 to 7 minutes or until the sauce is completely cooked and the flavours have blended. Lower the temperature.

- Assembling the enchiladas

- Turn the oven on high heat (350 degrees Fahrenheit) to start.

- Heat a flat pan or grill slightly on both sides to form the corn tortillas easily. The tortillas will be simpler to roll out as a result.

To form a stack, evenly divide the sweet potato and black bean mixture among the tortillas. After wrapping up the tortilla, place it seam-side down in a baking tray.

**Sauce Pour:** Evenly distribute the pre-made enchilada sauce over the covered enchiladas.

Before topping the enchiladas with vegan cheese, make sure it's properly distributed.

The enchiladas will be done, and the sauce will begin to bubble when you bake them in a preheated oven for 20 to 25 minutes.

Upon removing the enchiladas from the oven, garnish with sliced jalapenos and chopped cilantro. Reheat and present.

**Instructions:** Adjust the heat level of the meal by adjusting the amount of chilli powder and jalapenos according to your taste.

To make your enchiladas unique, include corn kernels, avocado slices, or sliced bell peppers in the mixture.

So that they don't contain gluten, you may cook these enchiladas using gluten-free corn tortillas.

I was reheating some delicious leftovers from the night before for another delicious dinner.

Sweet potato and black bean enchiladas have a wonderful texture and flavour combination thanks to the roasted sweet potatoes and the earthy richness of the black beans. A satisfying and nutritious vegan supper option, perfect for family dinners or social gatherings. Add some colour and flavour to your table with these enchiladas, which are luscious and flavorful. You may top them with some delicious tomato sauce and vegan cheese if you'd like.

**Chapter 7: Sides and Accompaniments**

- **Recipe 26: Roasted Garlic and Herb Cauliflower**

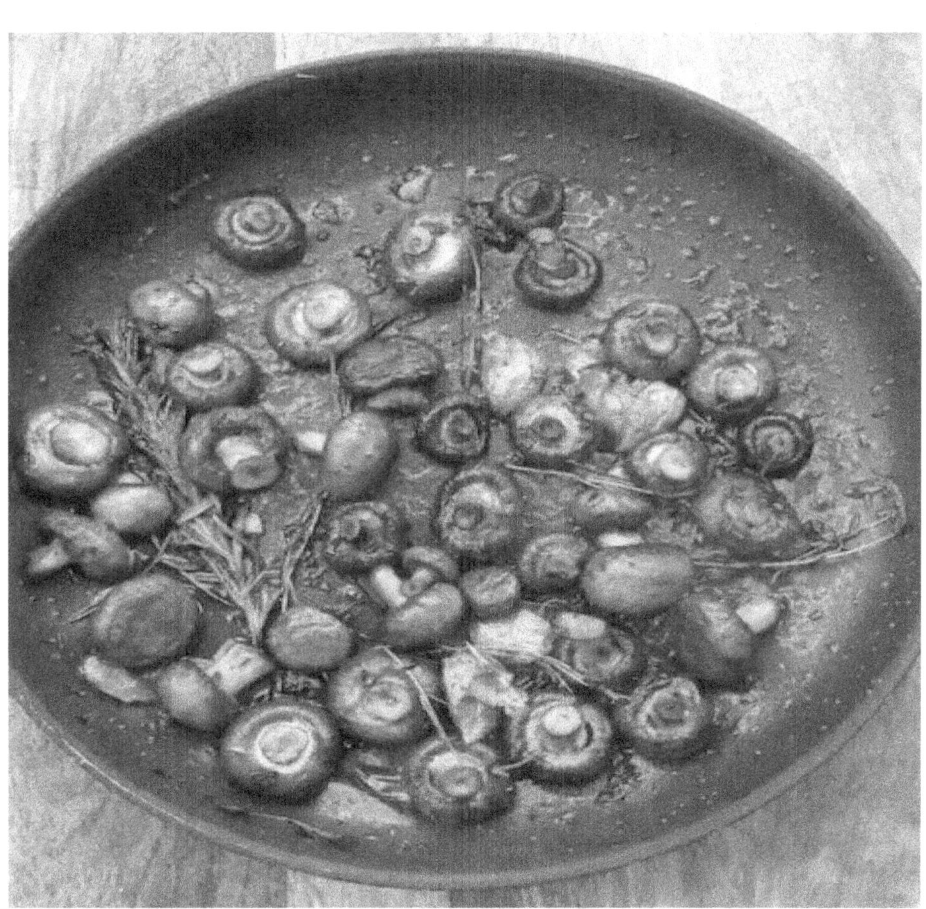

**Ingredients:**

One big head of cauliflower with small heads on it.

6 to 8 chopped garlic cloves that have been peeled

2 to 3 teaspoons of fresh herbs, chopped, like parsley, rosemary, or thyme

It has three teaspoons of olive oil.

One teaspoon of salt, or as much as you like

Add half a teaspoon of black pepper or more to taste.

The zest of one lemon may be left out for a more colorful garnish.

If you want it with a tart taste, drizzle in 1/4 to 1/2 teaspoon of lemon juice.

**Instructions:**

Cook until the temperature reaches 425 °F, or 220 degrees Celsius, with a rack lying in the center.

Cauliflower preparation involves giving the head a good wash and removing the stiff stalk and leaves. Make bite-sized florets out of it. For consistent cooking, make sure the florets are around the same size.

*Mince garlic:* Peel the garlic cloves and finely mince them.

*Herb blends:* A little bowl is all you need to combine fresh herbs like rosemary, parsley, or thyme with olive oil, salt, and black pepper. To create a delicious oil infused with herbs, combine all ingredients well.

**To coat cauliflower:**

1. Put the florets in a large mixing basin.

2. Pour the oil mixture flavored with herbs over the cauliflower, tossing to cover well.

3. Make sure that the fragrant mixture has covered every floret.

*Spread on Baking Sheet:* Put parchment paper over a baking sheet to make it easy to clean. Ensure that the cauliflower pieces are spread out evenly on the baking pan. In this way, you can be sure of a uniform roast and a beautiful brown color.

*Roast:* Place the baking sheet in an oven that has already been heated up. Roast the cauliflower for 25 to 30 minutes, or until it is soft to the touch and has a light, crispy, golden skin. To check if the florets are done, put a fork or stick into the largest part of one and slide it in easily.

*Optional Lemon Finish:* While the roasted cauliflower is still hot, you may add a zesty touch by dusting lemon zest on top. Add some additional lemon juice for an extra citrus taste boost.

Transfer the cauliflower with the roasted garlic and herbs to a serving tray or dish to be served. If desired, add more fresh herbs as a garnish.

*Enjoy:* Serving your roasted garlic and herb cauliflower as a delicious side dish with your favorite main dishes. It complements grilled tofu, roasted meats, and as a delicious accompaniment to a buffet of vegetables.

**Cooking Notes:**

You are welcome to alter the herb mixture to suit your tastes. Try combining herbs like rosemary and thyme for a traditional taste, or try other fresh herbs like oregano or sage.

Lemon zest and juice give the meal vibrancy and a sense of citrus, but you may omit them if you want a milder taste.

The cauliflower may be roasted until it is as soft as you want. While some want it more delicate and caramelized, others love it with a little crunch.

Refrigerated leftovers may be used for wraps, sandwiches, salads, grain bowls, and other dishes.

- **Recipe 27: Turmeric Rice**

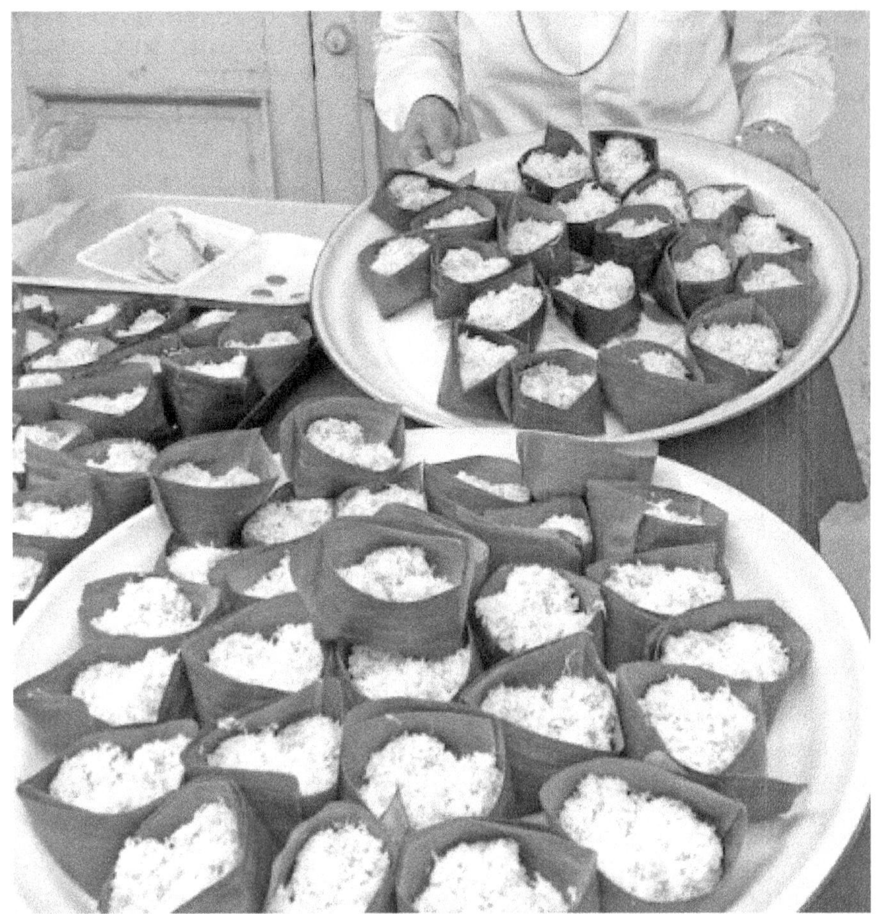

**Ingredients:**

Long-Grain White Rice: 1 cup (try Basmati rice for a lighter flavor).

Two cups of water

Half a teaspoon of turmeric powder

Olive oil or ghee: 2 teaspoons of

Please chop two to three garlic cloves.

One little onion, thinly sliced.

As much salt as you choose, up to half a teaspoon.

1/4 teaspoon black pepper, or more if you like it spicier

It's optional to add two tablespoons of chopped fresh cilantro.

**Lemon Zest: 1 lemon**

**Instructions:**

*Rice Rinse:* Rinse the rice well under cold running water to remove any debris. This removes any surplus starch and keeps the rice from becoming too sticky.

*Combine Water and Turmeric:* Two cups of water and half a teaspoon of turmeric powder should be combined in a saucepan. Stir the turmeric well to distribute it evenly. This is why the water is colored with brilliant yellow turmeric.

*Cook Rice with Turmeric Water:* Bring the water that has turmeric in it to a full boil. After the water has boiled, add the clean rice to the pot. Give the rice a quick spin to make sure it's spread out evenly. With the cover on for around fifteen to twenty minutes, cook the rice over low heat. Check the rice's package for cooking instructions, as times may vary.

Rice should be fluffed after it has finished cooking and the water has been absorbed. For approximately five minutes, let it sit covered. Then, separate the grains of rice by fluffing it with a fork. The rice will have a lovely golden hue because of the turmeric.

**Sauté Garlic and Onion:**

1. Melt the olive oil or ghee in a separate pan over medium heat.

2. Chop the onion finely and throw it in the pan. The onion should become translucent and slightly browned after three or four minutes of sautéing.

3. When the garlic begins to smell wonderful, add the chopped garlic and stir for one or two more minutes.

*Rice and Onion Mixture:* Put the cooked rice in the pan with the garlic, onion, and other spices. Mix well. The onion and garlic smells can now be taken in by the rice.

*Salt and pepper to taste:* Season the rice with turmeric and then add salt and black pepper. Boil the rice for two to three minutes and stir it around a lot to mix the tastes.

*Garnish:* You may add freshly chopped cilantro and lemon zest to the turmeric rice as a final touch. These additives give the dish a flavorful and fresh boost.

Put the turmeric rice on a tray or serving dish so it's ready to be served. Now it's ready to be made as a colorful and tasty side dish for many different kinds of main dishes.

**Cooking Notes:**

When sautéing the rice with the turmeric, you may add additional fragrant spices for a deeper flavor, such as cumin seeds, cardamom pods, or cinnamon sticks.

Increase the quantity of turmeric powder to your desired level if you like a stronger turmeric taste and color.

Various foods, including grilled chicken, fish, vegetarian curries, and stir-fries, go well with turmeric rice.

For further meals, leftover turmeric rice may be chilled and reheated. It can also be used in rice salads or stuffed inside bell peppers for a tasty variation.

- **Recipe 28: Roasted Root Vegetables**

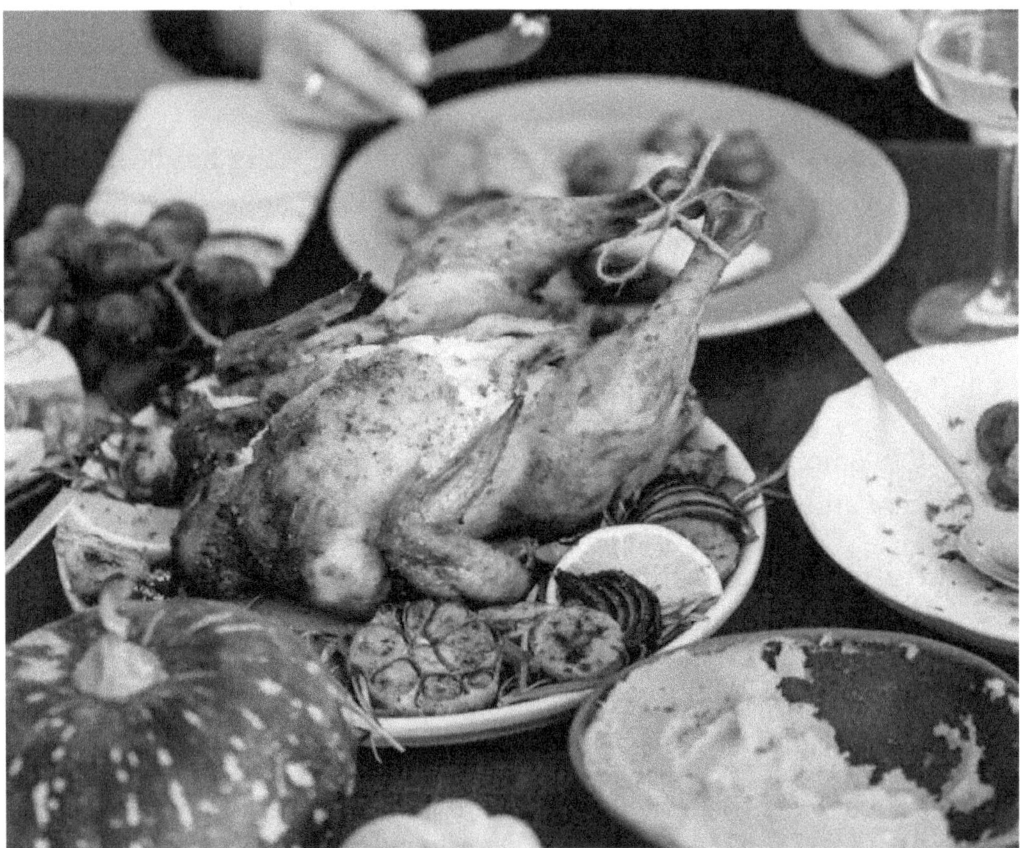

**Ingredients:**

Assorted Root Vegetables: Pick a selection that weighs between two and three pounds, including carrots, parsnips, sweet potatoes, turnips, and beets.

3–4 teaspoons of olive oil

1-2 sprigs each of rosemary and thyme (or your favorite herbs)

4-5 minced cloves of garlic

Half a teaspoon of black pepper, or more to taste, and one teaspoon of salt

Red onion slices, entire garlic cloves, or shallots as optional additions for taste

**Instructions:**

Turn on the oven and heat it to 425 degrees Fahrenheit (220 degrees Celsius). In the middle of the oven, you should put a rack.

How to Prepare the Vegetables: The root vegetables should be washed, peeled (if you want), and cut into uniform pieces that are about 1 inch cubes or chunks. Sizes that are all the same make cooking more even.

In a small saucepan, heat the olive oil over low heat for the garlic and herb decoction. Fresh thyme and rosemary leaves are also a good addition. Allow the garlic and leaves to steep in the heated oil for about five minutes. The aromas and flavors are released during this procedure.

In a large dish, combine the cooked root vegetables with the seasonings. Toss the veggies with the flavored olive oil and combine them. Salt and pepper would be great additions. Mix them to ensure the veggies are coated uniformly with the seasoned oil.

**Spread on Baking Sheet:**

1.  If you want your baking sheet to be simple to clean, line the bottom with parchment paper or a baking mat made of plastic.

2.  Spread out the seasoned root vegetables on a baking dish.

3.  Refrain from crowding people together since this may hinder even roasting.

Add salt and pepper to the root veggies and roast them in a preheated oven. Before roasting, give them 30 to 40 minutes. After 20 minutes, use a spoon to carefully flip the vegetables over so that they cook evenly. They should be roasted until the outside is browned and the inside is soft.

*Optional Additions:* During the last 15-20 minutes of roasting, you may add shallots, entire garlic cloves, or slices of red onion to the oven sheet. They'll develop a sweet, delicate flavor.

Remove the herb sprigs from the roasted root vegetables before serving as a garnish. Add more fresh herbs as a garnish for a splash of color and flavor.

Place the roasted root vegetables on a serving tray or dish to be served. They may now be savored as a delicious and calming side dish.

**Cooking Notes:**

You are welcome to alter the flavor by adding your preferred dry herbs or spices. A sprinkle of cayenne pepper, cumin, or paprika may provide some heat.

To suit your tastes, try out several root vegetable varieties. Yams, celery root, and rutabagas are other fantastic options.

Before roasting the veggies, drizzle them with honey, maple syrup, or a little brown sugar for a subtle sweetness.

You may use leftover roasted root vegetables in salads, grain bowls, or as a tasty side for subsequent meals by storing them in the refrigerator.

- **Recipe 29: Quinoa and Kale Pilaf**

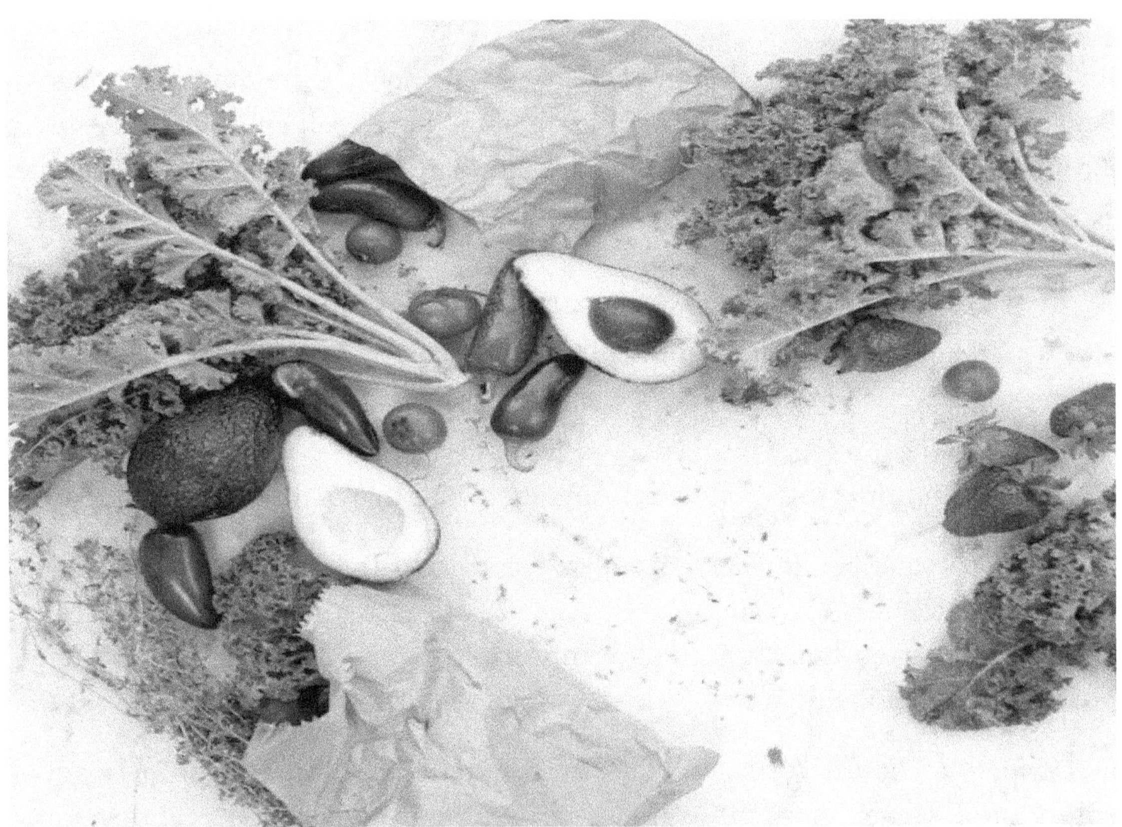

**Ingredients:**

1 cup of quinoa that has been cleaned and drained

To cook the quinoa, you'll need two cups of water or veggie broth.

One bunch of kale with the stems cut off and the leaves cut up.

Two milliliters of olive oil

One medium-sized onion, cut up small

Please chop two to three garlic cloves.

Two medium-sized carrots, cut up

One red bell pepper cut up.

One teaspoon of cumin seeds

A half teaspoon of powdered coriander

As much salt as you choose, up to half a teaspoon.

To taste, add 1/4 teaspoon of black pepper. more heat

Half a teaspoon of lemon juice

1/4 cup chopped toasted nuts (for decoration)

**Instructions:**
Before cooking quinoa, rinse it under cold water, often through a fine-mesh sieve. In doing so, you may remove the bitter coating.
**Quinoa and water:** Combine the rinsed quinoa with two cups of water or vegetable broth in a saucepan. Place the cover on top and reduce the heat to low. Cook, covered, for 15–20 minutes, or until quinoa is tender and the liquid has evaporated. Once the five minutes are up, please remove it from the heat, cover it, and allow it to rest for another five. Fluff with a fork.

**Kale and quinoa pilaf:**

*Sauté Garlic and Onion:*

Olive oil should be warmed in a large saucepan over medium heat.

Toss in the onion after dicing it. To make the onion translucent, sauté it for a couple of minutes.

When the garlic smells wonderful, add the chopped garlic and stir for one or two more minutes.

In chopped form, you should also add red bell pepper and carrots to the pan. If you sauté them for about 5 to 7 minutes, they should get soft.

Kale should be cooked after adding salt, black pepper, ground cumin, and coriander. To the skillet, add the chopped kale leaves. Sauté the kale for 3-5 minutes or until it wilts and softens.

***Combine Quinoa and Kale:*** Toss in the cooked quinoa with the sautéed vegetables and greens. Just give everything a little toss to heat it all.

***Lemon Juice to Finish:*** Add lemon juice to the quinoa and kale pilaf and combine. The meal gets a revitalizing punch from the lemon juice.

Top the pilaf with finely chopped, roasted almonds to add crunch and taste.

Move the kale and quinoa rice to a bowl or plate for serving. Serve hot. As a tasty and healthy main dish or side food, it is ready to be served.

**Cooking Notes:**

You may add different veggies like peas, corn, or chopped tomatoes to add more color and nutrients to the pilaf.

To suit your preferences, experiment with various seasonings. Add a little red pepper flakes or chili powder for a hotter variation.

Use vegetable broth or water to cook the quinoa, and omit the optional toasted almonds for garnish if you want to make this recipe vegan.

Refrigerated leftovers may be eaten for lunch or supper the following day or used as stuffing for wraps or stuffed peppers.

- **Recipe 30: Cucumber and Tomato Salad**

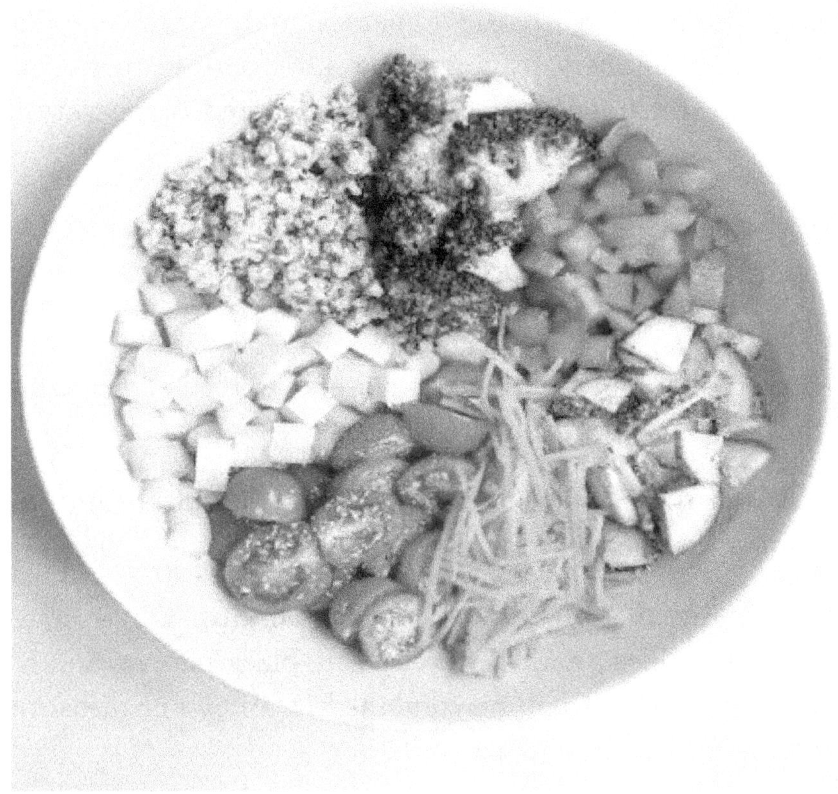

**Ingredients:**

Two large cucumbers or three or four smaller ones should be thinly sliced.

Three to four tiny tomatoes, diced, or two large ones

Feel free to add one thinly sliced little red onion if you choose.

Substitute 1/4 cup of chopped fresh parsley or cilantro for the 1/4 cup of fresh basil.

Half a cup of crumbled feta cheese is optional.

Three tablespoons of olive oil are in it.

Substitute balsamic vinegar for the red wine vinegar if you like a sweeter flavor.

As much salt as you choose, up to half a teaspoon.

One-fourth teaspoon of black pepper, or more to taste

(Optional) 1 or 2 cloves of chopped garlic (for flavor)

A tablespoon of honey (or more, depending on your preference)

**Instructions:**

*Vegetable preparation:* Thoroughly wash the tomatoes and cucumbers. You may completely or partly peel the cucumbers, leaving some skin on for texture. Cucumbers are cut into small slices, and tomatoes are diced. Slice your red onion very thinly if you're using it.

Sliced cucumbers, diced tomatoes, and thinly sliced red onion (if used) should all be combined in a large mixing basin. Your cucumber and tomato salad's foundation is created in this way.

Sprinkle the chopped fresh basil (or any herbs you choose) over the veggies to add fresh herbs. The herbs give the dish a flavorful and fresh boost.

Feta cheese is optional; scatter some over the salad if you use it. The creamy and tangy flavor of the feta cheese enhances the crisp veggies.

*Dressing Preparation:* Make the dressing in a separate, small dish. Olive oil, red wine vinegar (or balsamic vinegar), minced garlic (if used), salt, black pepper, and honey (if you'd like a touch of sweetness) should all be combined in a bowl or measuring cup. Use a whisk to mix the dressing's parts together well.

*Salad:* Add the sauce to the tomato and cucumber salad and mix it all together. To make sure the vegetables are all covered in the sauce, use two big spoons or salad tongs to gently toss everything together.

*Shake:* Allow the salad to chill for at least 30 minutes before serving. Wrap the bowl in plastic or place a lid on top. Chilling the salad enhances its flavor and adds a refreshing twist to its taste.

The cucumber and tomato salad is ready to be served after it has cooled. It makes a delicious side dish for barbecues and picnics and is a light and healthful addition to any dinner.

**Cooking Notes:**

To add more variation and taste to this salad, add more items like olives, red or yellow bell peppers, or pieces of avocado.

You may alter the dressing by varying the honey, vinegar, or garlic amounts.

Although this salad may be served immediately, chilling it in the refrigerator makes it even more delectable.

Save any leftovers in a sealed container and store them in the fridge for up to two days. Before serving, give it a good spin to revive the flavors.

**Chapter 8: Sauces and Dressings**

- **Recipe 31: Turmeric Tahini Dressing**

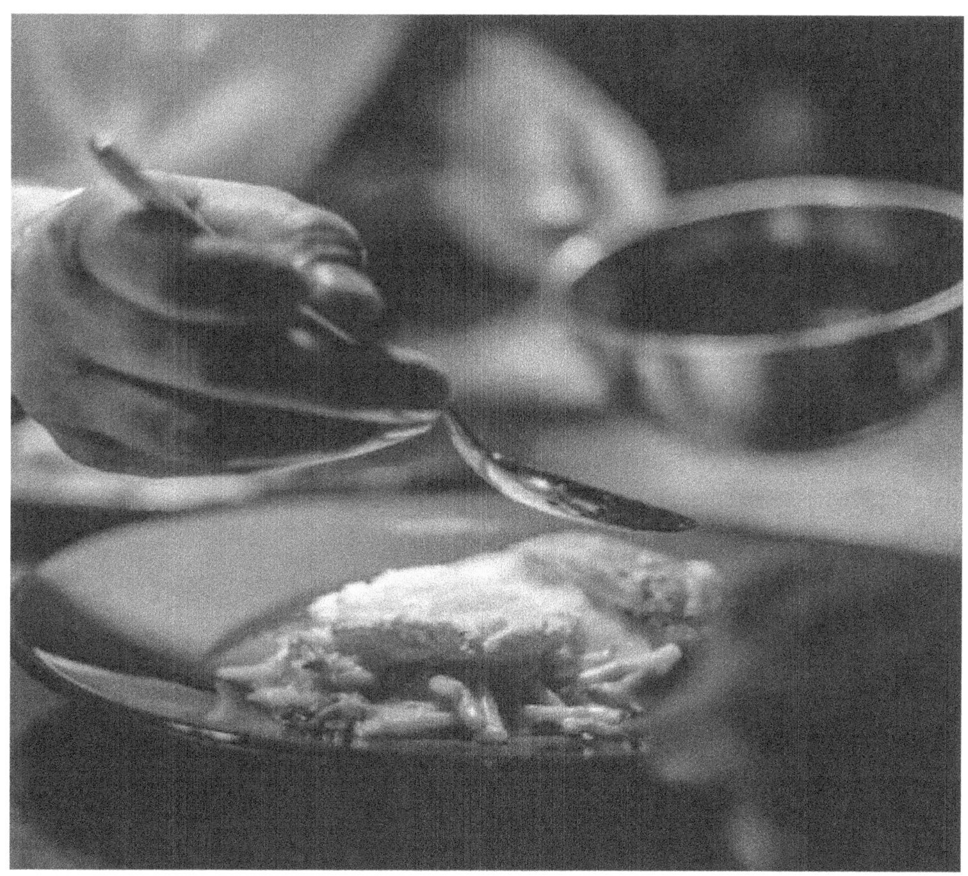

Ingredients:

Ingredients: 1/4 cup of tahini, a sesame seed paste.

In place of 2 teaspoons of lemon juice that has just been squeezed

Add 2–3 teaspoons of water (or more or less for taste).

Cumin powder, half a teaspoon

0.5 teaspoons of cumin powder ground coriander, half a teaspoon. For more flavor, add one minced tiny clove.

**A half teaspoon of mineral salt**

**Black pepper, 1/4 teaspoon**

**Two teaspoons of olive oil that is extra-virgin for added sweetness**

**Use one or two tablespoons of honey or maple syrup**

**Instructions:**

1. *Combine Tahini and Juice from the lemon fruit:* Mix the lemon juice that has just been squeezed with the tahini in a mixing dish. What you're making here is the creamy base for your turmeric tahini sauce.

2. *Add Water:* Slowly add two to three tablespoons of water to the tahini and lemon mix. How much water you use will depend on how thick or thin you want your dressing to be. If you want the sauce to be thinner, add more water. If you want it to be thicker, add less water. Mix the ingredients together with a whisk until the mixture is smooth.

3. *Incorporate Spices:* Mix in the ground cumin, coriander, salt, black pepper, chopped garlic (if using), and turmeric powder. These spices give turmeric tahini sauce its unique golden color and a burst of flavor.

4. *Blend Well:* Whisk the dressing vigorously until the spices are fully incorporated into the tahini mixture. Ensure there are no lumps and the dressing is smooth and homogeneous.

5. *Add Olive Oil:* While the sauce is still being mixed, add the extra-virgin olive oil. The dressing tastes rich and spicy thanks to the olive oil, which makes it creamier.

6. *Sweeten (Optional):* Add 1-2 teaspoons of maple syrup or honey if you prefer a slightly sweet dressing. Sweetener is optional, and you can adjust the amount to your taste.

7. *Taste and Adjust:* Taste the sauce and change the spices before serving. To get the taste you want, add salt, pepper, lemon juice, or a sweetener.

8. *Store or Serve:* The turmeric tahini dressing can be kept in the fridge for up to a week in a jar that won't let air in. Before you use it, please stir it well. You can also use it right away as a dipping sauce for different foods or as a delicious dressing for salads, roasted veggies, and grain bowls.

**Recipe Notes:**

- Many different things may be made using turmeric tahini sauce. Fresh herbs, such as cilantro, parsley or hot red pepper flakes, might change the flavor profile.

- If the sauce gets thicker in the fridge, add more water to change the consistency. And when it gets cold, the olive oil can harden. If this happens, let the dressing warm up to room temperature before using it.

- Experiment with this dressing as a marinade for grilled vegetables, tofu, or chicken for a delightful flavor boost.

- Turmeric imparts a vibrant color and offers potential health benefits due to its anti-inflammatory properties. Enjoy this dressing as a nutritious and flavorful addition to your meals.

- **Recipe 32: Basil Pesto with Walnuts**

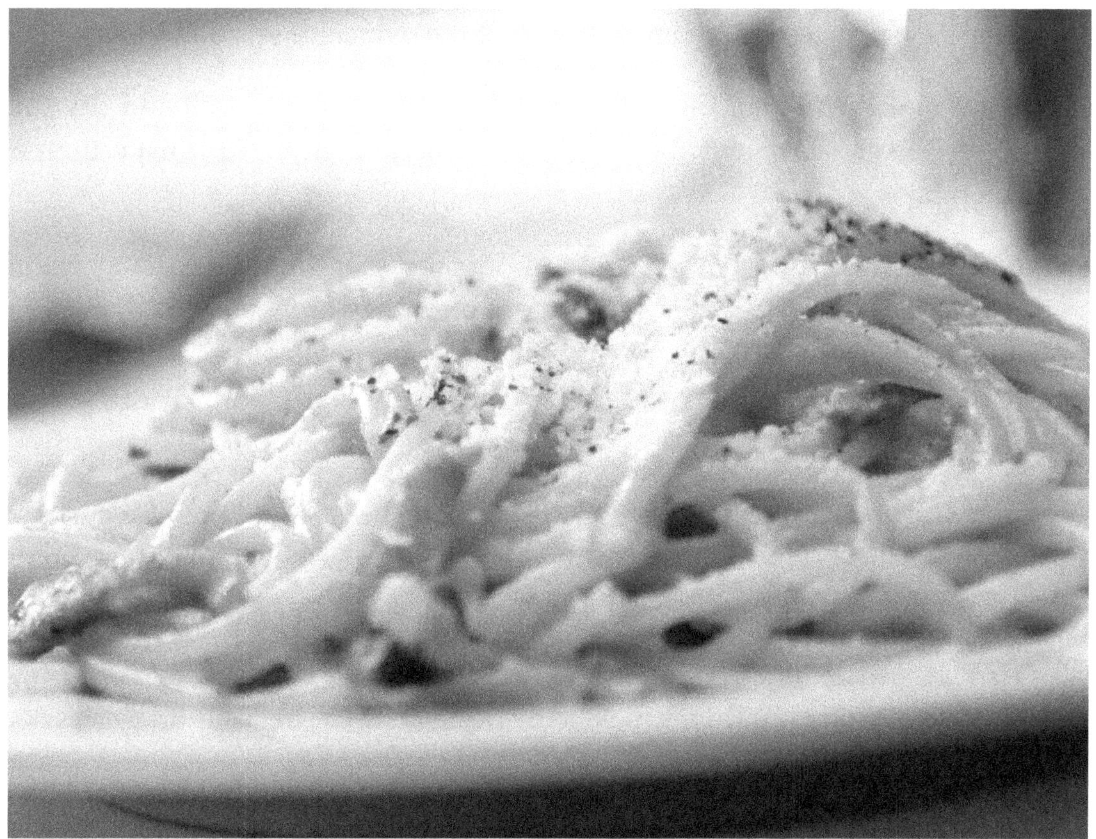

**Ingredients:**

- **Fresh Basil Leaves:** 2 cups, packed

- **Walnuts:** 1/2 cup, toasted

- **Garlic Cloves:** 2-3 cloves, minced

- **Parmesan Cheese:** Grate 1/2 cup of cheese (Pecorino Romano for a spicier taste).

- **Lemon Juice:** 2 tablespoons, freshly squeezed

- **Olive oil that is 100% pure: 1/2 cup**

- **A half teaspoon of mineral salt**

- **one-fourth teaspoon of black pepper**

**Instructions:**

1. *Toast Walnuts:* To get the oven to 175°F or 350°F, preheat it. Arrange the walnuts on a baking pan in a single layer. Toast them in a preheated oven for 5–7 minutes or until fragrant and slightly brown. Make sure they don't become too hot by keeping a close eye on them. Take out of the oven and let cool.

2. *Wash and Prep Basil:* Clean the fresh basil leaves really well and dry them with paper towels. Take out the tough stems because they can make the pesto less smooth.

3. *Combine Basil and Walnuts:* In a food processor, mix the toasted walnuts and fresh basil leaves together. Pulse them until they are well mixed and broken up into small pieces. To ensure that all the ingredients are processed in the same manner, you may need to carefully remove any food debris from the bowl of the food processor.

4. *Add Garlic and Cheese:* Grate the Parmesan cheese and chop the garlic and add them to the basil and walnuts in the food processor. Once more, pulse until everything is well mixed.

5. *Drizzle Lemon Juice:* While the food processor is going, slowly add the newly squeezed lemon juice. This makes the pesto taste fresher and bright.

6. *Stream in Olive Oil:* Whirl the extra-virgin olive oil slowly through the feed tube of the running food processor. Keep processing the pesto until it has the consistency you want. Some people like their pesto smooth, while others like it with a few chunks. You can change how much olive oil you use to get the thickness you want.

7. ***Add pepper and salt:*** Put the blender down and sample some pesto. Season with salt and pepper to taste. get the desired level of seasoning.

8. ***Serve or Store:*** Put the basil pesto in a container or jar that won't let air in. If you want to use it right away, it's ready to be a tasty pasta sauce, a sandwich spread, or a topping for meats and veggies on the grill. If you want to store the pesto for up to a week, To prevent spoilage, drizzle a thin coating of olive oil over it. For even longer storage, try freezing it in ice cube trays.

**Recipe Notes:**

- You can customize your basil pesto by adding other ingredients like pine nuts, almonds, or pecans for a unique twist on flavor and texture.

- Skip the Parmesan cheese or use a dairy-free cheese instead if you want to make this pesto meatless. You can also get a cheesy taste without the dairy by using nutritional yeast.

- Experiment with the pesto by adding sun-dried tomatoes, roasted red peppers, or spinach for different variations.

- This homemade basil pesto offers fresh, aromatic flavors and can elevate various dishes, from pasta to bruschetta to grilled chicken. Enjoy its vibrant taste and versatility in your culinary creations.

- **Recipe 33: Ginger Soy Glaze**

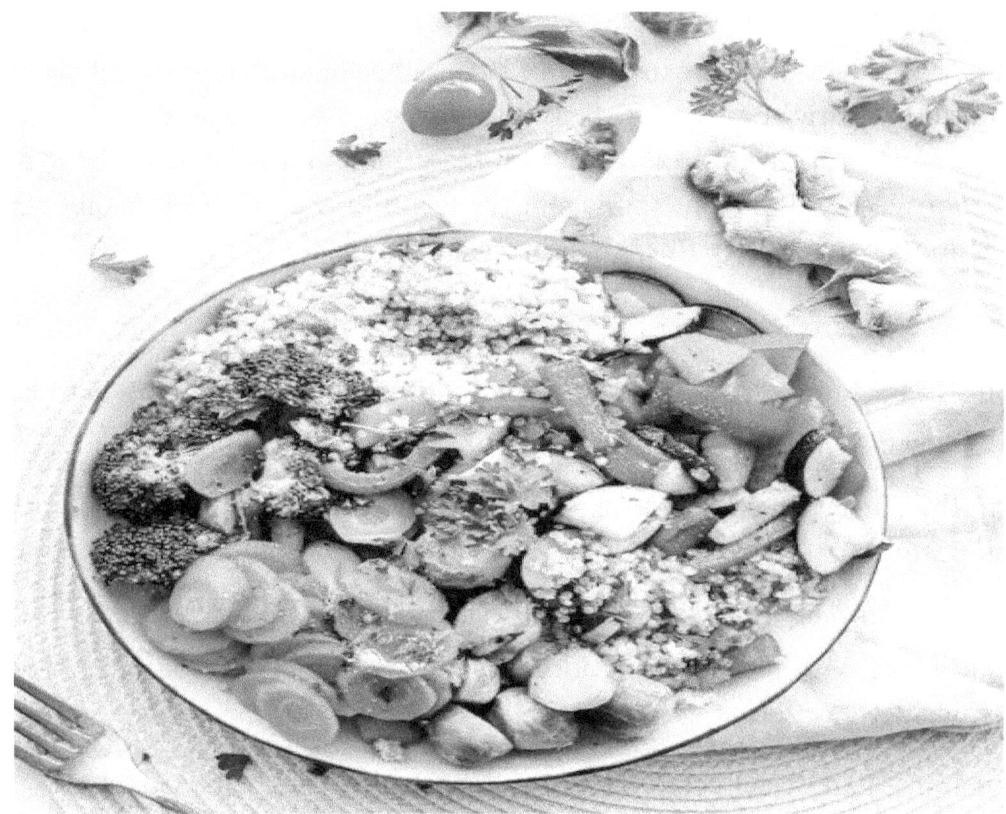

Ingredients:

- 1/2 cup of soy sauce (any kind would do, although a low-sodium one is ideal)

- The quantity of brown sugar may be adjusted to your preference.

- minced garlic, and two teaspoons of fresh ginger. One minced clove of cloves

- Rice If you want, you may substitute apple cider vinegar for the vinegar.

- You may optionally add 1 teaspoon of sesame oil for a nutty flavor.

- To thicken, if desired, add 1 tablespoon of cornstarch.

- How much water will you require? Two tablespoons

- If you're looking for a little heat, add 1/2 teaspoon of red pepper flakes.

- Two or three thin slices of green onion (for garnishing purposes, if preferred)

Instructions:

1. ***Combine Soy Sauce and Sugar:*** First, combine the brown sugar and soy sauce in a small saucepan. While cooking over medium-low heat, stir the mixture to dissolve the sugar. This is the foundation for your spicy and sweet ginger soy sauce.

2. ***Add Ginger and Garlic:*** Cut the garlic clove into small pieces and grate the fresh ginger. Put them both in the pan with the soy sauce and sugar. To mix the tastes, stir them well.

3. ***Incorporate Vinegar and Optional Sesame Oil:*** Pour in the rice vinegar (or apple cider vinegar) and add the sesame oil if you use it. These ingredients add a tangy and nutty dimension to the glaze. Stir to combine.

4. ***Create Cornstarch Slurry (Optional):*** One tablespoon of cornstarch and two tablespoons of water mixed together in a separate small bowl will make the glaze thicker. This will help make the glaze as thick as you want it to be.

5. ***Thicken the Glaze:*** If you've prepared the cornstarch slurry, pour it into the saucepan with the other ingredients. Stir the glaze continuously over medium heat until it thickens. This usually takes 1-2 minutes. If you prefer a thinner glaze, you can skip this step.

6. ***Add Optional Red Pepper Flakes:*** If you'd like to add some heat to your ginger soy glaze, sprinkle in the red pepper flakes. Adjust the amount to your preferred level of spiciness.

7. ***Taste and Adjust:*** You can change the flavor of the glaze to suit your tastes. You can make it sweeter by adding more sugar, salty by adding soy sauce, or sour by adding vinegar.

8. ***Cool and Serve:*** Take the ginger soy sauce off the heat and let it cool down. It will get a little thicker as it cools. It's ready to serve after it cools down.

9. ***Garnish (Optional):*** Garnish the glaze with finely sliced green onions for a fresh and colorful touch.

10. ***Serve:*** Use the ginger soy glaze as a flavorful drizzle over grilled meats, seafood, vegetables, or rice. It also makes a delicious dipping sauce for spring rolls, dumplings, or sushi.

**Recipe Notes:**

- This ginger soy glaze is highly versatile and can be used in various Asian-inspired dishes. It perfectly balances sweet, salty, tangy, and savory flavors.

- You can change the amounts and items to fit your taste. You can add more sugar if you want it sweeter or less soy sauce if you want it less salty.

- Any extra sauce can be kept in the fridge for up to a week in a jar that won't let air in. Warm it up slowly on the stove or in the microwave before you use it.

- **Recipe 34: Avocado Cilantro Lime Sauce**

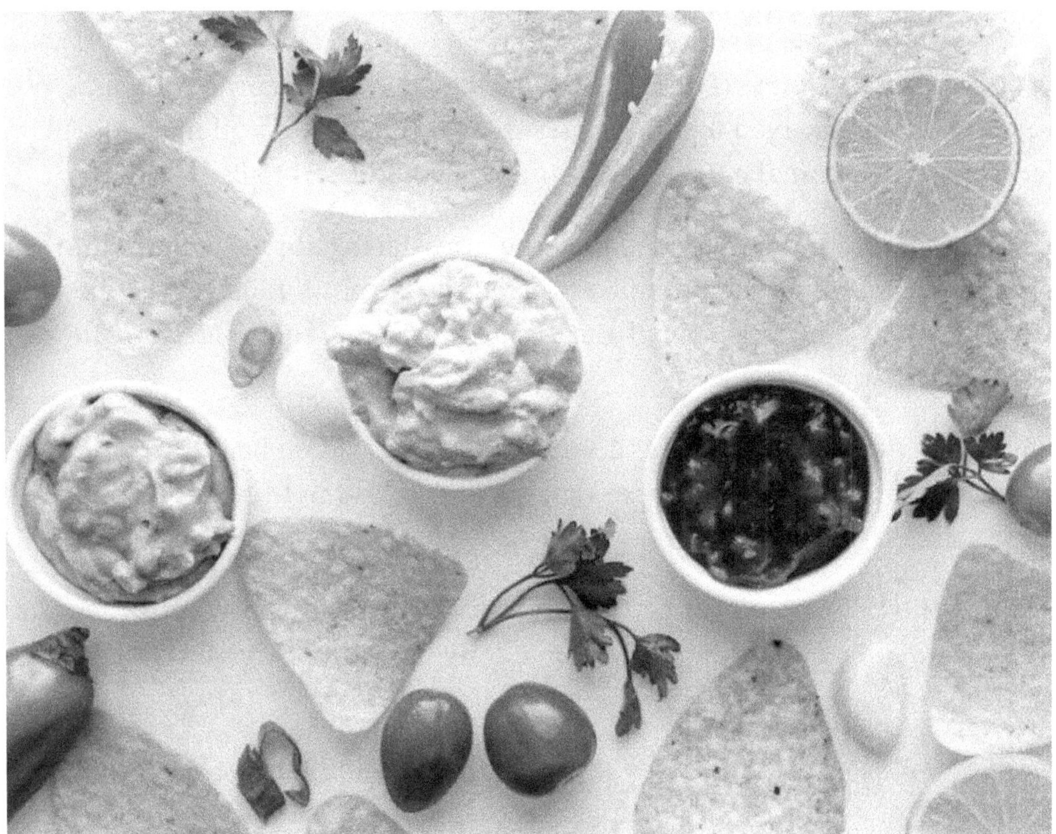

**Ingredients:**

- **A single ripe avocado, halved and seeded**

- **To taste, adjust the quantity of chopped fresh cilantro to 1/2 cup.**

- **Lime juice: 2 limes, plus or less, as desired.**

- **Cloves for Bok Choy: one clove, finely chopped**

- **If you want it creamier, add 1/4 cup of Greek yogurt.**

- **Two teaspoons of olive oil that is extra-virgin**

- **A half teaspoon of mineral salt**

- **Black pepper, 1/4 teaspoon**

- **For spiciness, add 1/4 teaspoon of red pepper flakes.**

- **Water: 2–4 tablespoons (adjust according to taste)**

**Instructions:**

1. *Prepare Avocado:* Take the pit out of the ripe avocado and cut it in half. Then, put the meat into a blender or food processor. For the creamiest results, make sure you use a ripe avocado.

2. *Add Cilantro:* Clean the fresh cilantro and cut it up. Put it in the mixer or food processor with the avocado.

3. *Squeeze Lime Juice:* Put the avocado, cilantro, and the juice of two limes into a blender or food processor. Change how much lime juice you use to get the level of sourness you like.

4. *Incorporate Minced Garlic:* For the garlic clove, chop it up and add it to the food in the blender or food processor.

5. *Optional Greek Yogurt:* Blend or process Greek yogurt if you want the sauce to be creamier. Adding Greek yogurt to the sauce makes it creamier without changing how fresh it is.

6. *Drizzle Olive Oil:* Blend or mix the food with the extra-virgin olive oil. For a thick and smooth sauce, this is added.

7. *Season with Salt and Pepper:* For extra flavor, add black pepper and salt. Red pepper flakes can be added now if you want it a little hotter.

8. *Blend Until Smooth:* Throw all of the sauce's components into a food processor. or blender and pulse until smooth and thick. Gradually add water and a tablespoon spoonful until the sauce reaches the desired consistency if it is too thick. Add the water again by blending.

9. *Taste and Adjust:* You may adjust the saltiness of the avocado cilantro lime sauce to your liking. Add more lime juice for a tangier taste. To taste, add more salt and pepper or water as required to adjust flavor.

10. *Serve:* Move the sauce to a bowl or other container for serving. After being chilled, it's now ready to be served as a tasty and cool side dish.

**Recipe Notes:**

- Customize the sauce by adjusting the ingredients to your taste. If you love cilantro, add more for a stronger cilantro flavor. Likewise, adjust the amount of garlic, lime juice, and Greek yogurt based on your preferences.

- You can dress a salad with this sauce, dip chips or vegetables in it, put it on grilled meats or fish, or drizzle it on tacos and wraps.

- If you have sauce left over, you can keep it in the fridge for one or two days in a sealed container. Press plastic wrap directly onto the sauce's surface before closing the jar to keep it from turning brown.

- Avocado cilantro lime sauce is delicious and a healthy addition to your meals. It offers the creaminess of avocado, the freshness of cilantro and lime, and the tanginess of Greek yogurt if you choose to include it. Enjoy its vibrant flavors!

- **Recipe 35: Anti-Inflammatory Vinaigrette**

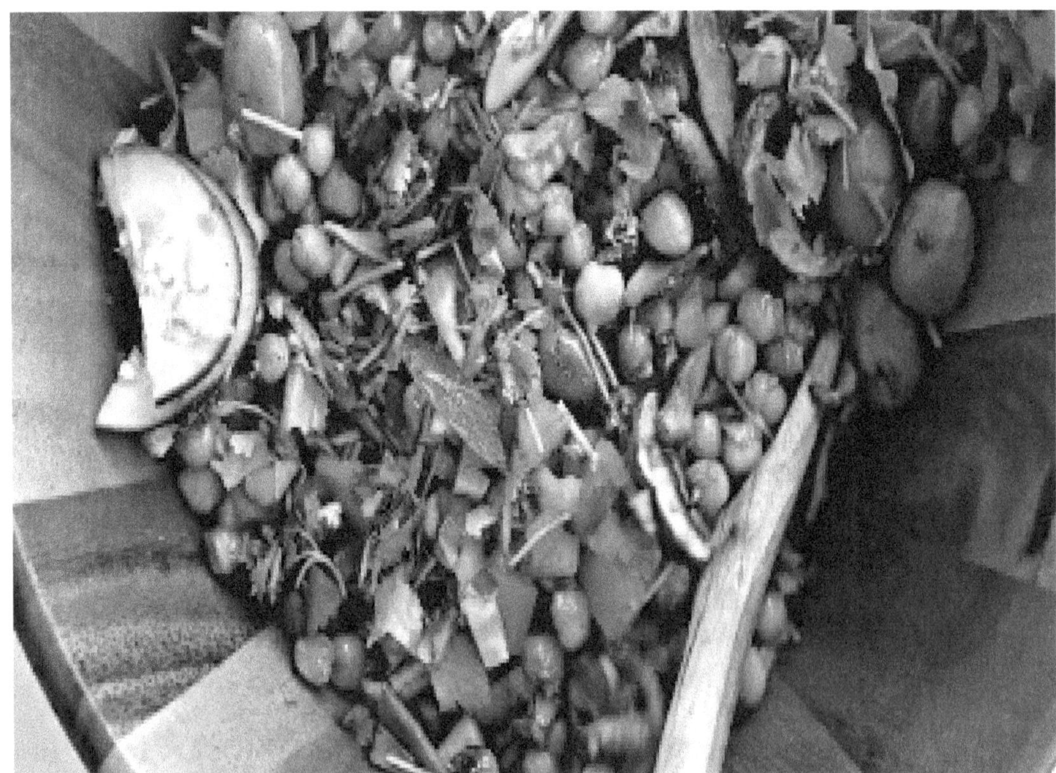

**Ingredients:**

- **The purest kind of olive oil: Half a cup**

- **Apple cider consumption of one-fourth cup of vinegar (preferably with the "mother" for added health benefits)**

- **Two teaspoons of honey (do a taste test)**

- **You need one teaspoon of turmeric powder, an anti-inflammatory spice.**

- **Another spice that aids in inflammation reduction is ground ginger, which requires 1/2 teaspoon.**

- **For a tart and creamy flavor, use 1 tablespoon of Dijon mustard.**

- **One minced garlic clove is all you need.**

- **Just under half a teaspoon of salt**

- **An eighth of a teaspoon of pepper**

**Instructions:**

1. *Bring together Olive Oil and Apple Cider Vinegar:* Very good olive oil and apple cider vinegar should be mixed together in a glass or non-reactive bowl. This is the base of your dressing that fights inflammation.

2. *Add Honey:* Add the honey all at once. The vinegar is sour, and the turmeric and ginger are spicy. The honey adds a little sweetness to balance it out.

3. *Incorporate Turmeric and Ginger:* Put the ground ginger and turmeric powder into the mix. People know that these two spices can help reduce inflammation. In addition, they give the dressing its bright color and taste.

4. Blend in Dijon Mustard: Add the Dijon mustard and mix well. Dijon mustard not only gives the dressing a sour kick, but it also helps the ingredients mix together, making the dressing smooth.

5. *Minced Garlic (Optional):* Try adding some minced garlic to give the vinaigrette a little more depth of flavor. Adding garlic, well-known for its health benefits, enhances the dressing's flavor.

6. *Add pepper and salt:* Toss in the salt and black pepper. Swap out the spices to get the desired flavor and level of saltiness.

7. ***Whisk Thoroughly:*** Whisk the vinaigrette vigorously until all the ingredients are well combined and the dressing has emulsified into a smooth and creamy texture.

8. ***Taste and Adjust:*** You can change the flavors of the anti-inflammatory dressing to suit your tastes. For more sweetness, vinegar for more tang, or spice for more heat, you can add more honey.

9. ***Store or Serve:*** Transfer the vinaigrette to an airtight container or glass jar. It's ready to drizzle over salads, roasted vegetables, or grilled proteins if you're using it immediately. If storing, keep it in the refrigerator for up to a week. Remember to give it a good shake or stir before each use to re-emulsify the ingredients.

**Recipe Notes:**

- You can change the dressing to fit your tastes. For more sweetness, add more honey. For more sourness, add more vinegar. You can change how much turmeric and ginger you use to get a softer or stronger taste.

- This anti-inflammatory vinaigrette can be used as a healthy and flavorful dressing for various dishes, promoting taste and wellness.

- Try experimenting with the vinaigrette by adding fresh herbs like cilantro and basil or a splash of citrus juice like lemon or orange for extra taste and nutrients.

- Embrace the benefits of this vinaigrette as part of an anti-inflammatory diet, and enjoy its vibrant and healing properties.

- **Recipe 36: Blueberry and Almond Oat Bars**

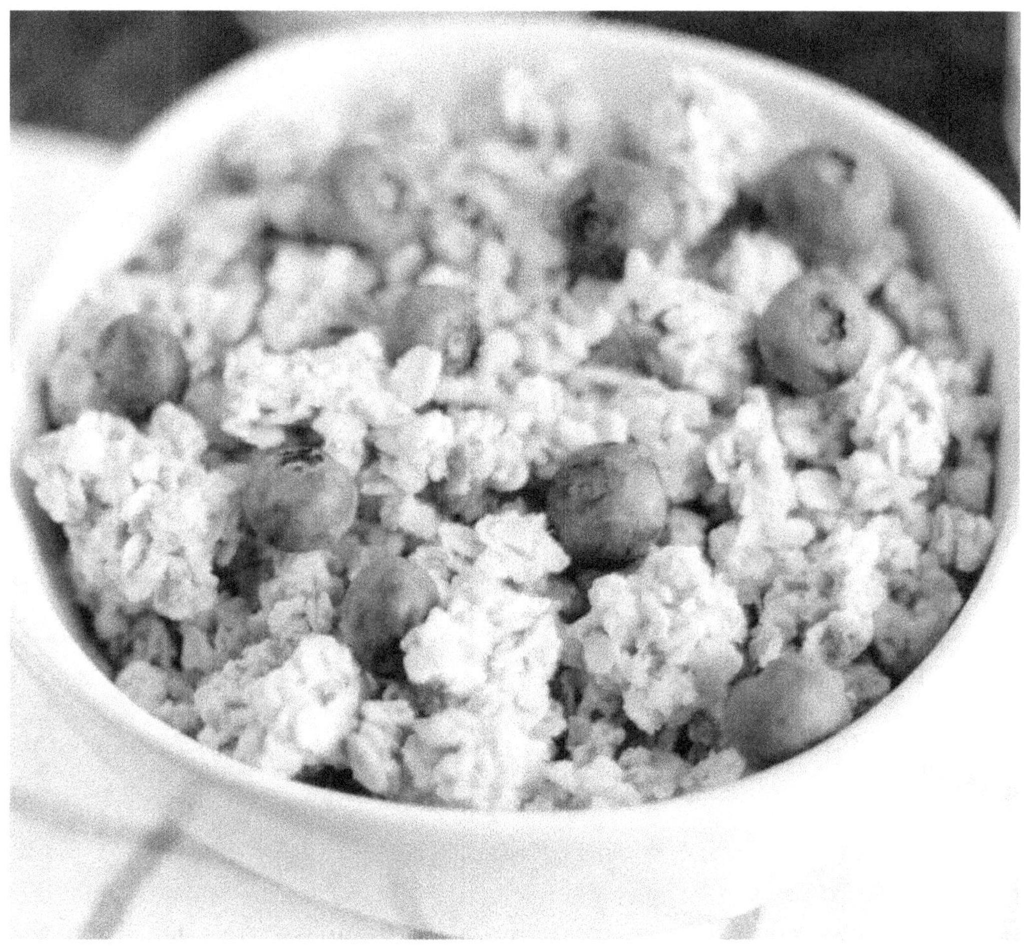

**Ingredients:**

For the Oat Base and Crumble:

- **A classic look Two cups of rolled oats**

- **Apple Almond One cup of flour**

- **Butter without salt: 1 stick (1/2 cup) melted**

- **To taste, add more honey if you want.**

- **One teaspoon of vanilla extract**

- **one-fourth teaspoon of salt**

**Regarding the Blueberry Curd:**

- **Blueberries:** two cups of fresh or frozen

- **Lemon Juice:** 2 tablespoons (freshly squeezed)

- **Granulated Sugar:** 1/4 cup (adjust to taste)

- **Cornstarch:** 2 tablespoons

**Instructions:**

*For the Oat Base and Crumble:*

1. *Get the oven ready:* Warm the oven up to 175°F (350°F). A 9x9-inch (23x23 cm) baking pan should be greased or lined with parchment paper, leaving some overflow to make it easy to take off.

2. *Combine Dry Ingredients:* Old-fashioned rolled oats, almond flour, and salt Combine everything in a large basin. Mix them well by stirring them together.

3. *Add Wet Ingredients:* Pour the honey, vanilla extract, and warmed unsalted butter into the pan. Mix the items together until they are well mixed. The mix should look like crumbled dough.

4. *Set Aside a Portion:* Save about two and a half to three cups of this oat mix. This is what will be used to finish the crumble.

**For the Blueberry Filling:**

1. *Prepare Blueberries:* If you are using frozen blueberries, let them thaw and squeeze out as much liquid as you can. If using fresh blueberries, rinse and pat them dry. Combine the blueberries with the lemon juice, granulated sugar, and cornstarch in a separate dish. Toss the berries to coat them well.

**Assembly:**

1. *Press the Oat Base:* The big piece of the oat mixture should be pressed evenly into the bottom of the baking pan that has been prepared. Make a hard, level base with your fingers or the back of a spoon.

2. *Add Blueberry Filling:* Spread the prepared filling evenly over the oat base.

3. *Crumble Topping:* Sprinkle the reserved oat mixture (the 1/2 to 2/3 cup you set aside) evenly over the blueberry filling. This forms the crumbly top layer.

4. *Bake:* Once the blueberry filling begins to boil and the top turns a golden brown, place the pan in the oven and bake for 35 to 40 minutes.

5. *Cool:* Allow the pan to cool on a wire rack following removing it from the oven. The bars must be chilled for them to solidify.

6. ***Slice and Serve:*** When the bars are totally cool, use the extra piece of parchment paper to lift them out of the pan. Cut them into squares or circles after putting them on a cutting board.

7. *Store:* If you have food left over, put it in a container that won't let air in. Leave it out at room temperature for one or two days, or put it in the fridge for longer. You can also freeze these bars and eat them later.

**Recipe Notes:**

- You can customize these oat bars by adding chopped nuts, seeds, or a dash of cinnamon to the oat mixture for added texture and flavor.

- Adjust the sweetness of the bars by increasing or decreasing the amount of honey or sugar in the blueberry filling to suit your taste.

- These bars make for a delightful breakfast or snack, offering a balance of wholesome oats, blueberries' natural sweetness, and almond flour's nutty richness. Enjoy them as a tasty and satisfying treat!

- Recipe 37: Dark Chocolate Avocado Mousse

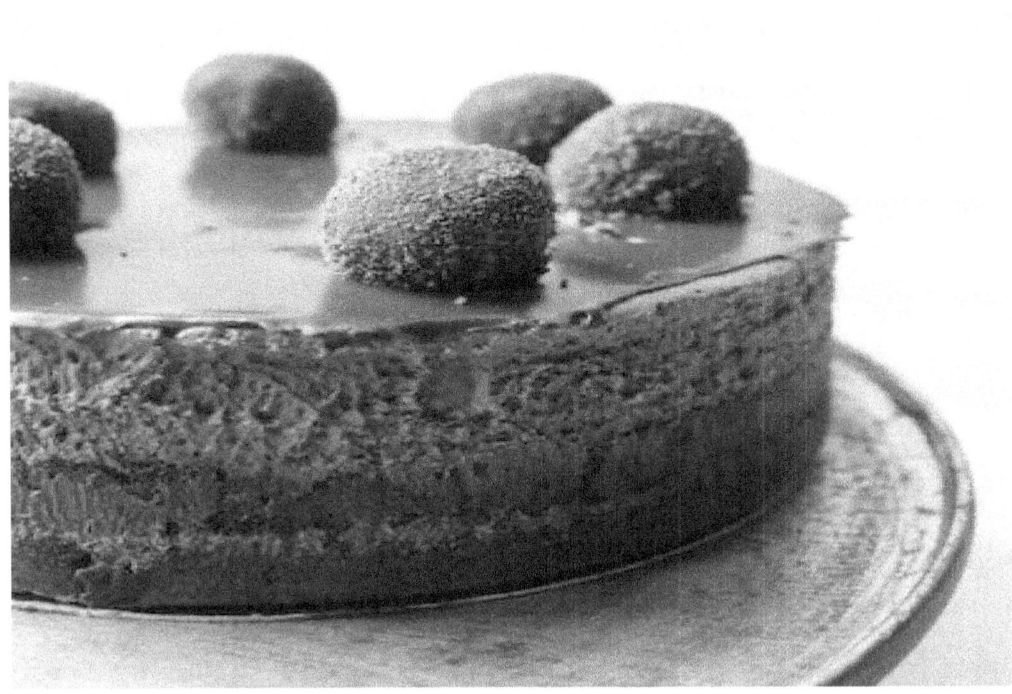

Ingredients:

- Two big avocados, de-pitted and skinned, when ripe

- Three and a half ounces (or 100 grams) of melted and cooled dark chocolate (with a cocoa content of 70% or greater for a richer taste)

- Unsweetened cocoa powder, 1/4 cup

- 1/4 cup maple syrup or honey (or use to your liking).

- Vanilla essence, measuring one teaspoon

- one-fourth teaspoon of salt

- Use fresh berries (strawberries, raspberries, etc.) as a garnish.

- Optional garnish: whipped cream

Instructions:

1. ***Melt the Dark Chocolate:*** First, melt the dark chocolate. Putting it in a bowl that can go in the microwave and cooking it for 15 seconds at a time while stirring it will melt it all. You could also use a double pot on the stove instead. After it melts, put it somewhere to cool down a bit.

2. ***Blend Avocado:*** In a food processor or high-speed mixer, mix the avocados that have been peeled and seeded together. Mix them together until they are smooth and creamy.

3. ***Add Dark Chocolate:*** Add the melted dark chocolate to the avocado that has been mixed. To keep the avocado from getting cooked, make sure the chocolate is not too hot. Once more, blend the chocolate and avocado together until they are completely mixed. This will make the texture rich and smooth.

4. ***Incorporate Cocoa Mass Powder:*** Toss in the unsweetened cocoa powder. Blend until the cocoa is thoroughly incorporated, giving the mousse its deep chocolate flavor.

5. ***Sweeten with Honey or Maple Syrup:*** Pour the vanilla extract on top of the honey or maple syrup. Mix it again until the sugar and vanilla are spread out evenly in the mousse. Check the sweetness and make changes as needed.

6. ***Season with Salt:*** Add a pinch of salt, which makes the chocolate taste better. Blend for a short time to mix.

7. ***Chill:*** Put the dark chocolate avocado mousse in a big bowl or individual serving plates. Cover with plastic wrap, making sure it touches the mousse's surface to keep it from going bad. Put it in the fridge for at least one to two hours to let the flavors mix and the mousse set.

8. ***Garnish:*** If you want, you can decorate the mousse with fresh berries (like strawberries or raspberries) and whipped cream before serving.

9. ***Serve:*** Serve your dark chocolate avocado mousse as a dessert or treat yourself to something nice. Take a bite of this sweet, creamy goodness.

**Recipe Notes:**

- For more taste, you can make your dark chocolate avocado mousse your own by adding a pinch of cinnamon, a splash of espresso, or a shot of your favorite liquor, like Grand Marnier or Amaretto.

- In addition to being delicious, this dish is also very healthy because it is full of avocados, which are high in healthy fats and fiber. Indulging in healthy ingredients in a tasty way will please your sweet tooth.

- If you have leftovers, you can keep them in the fridge for one or two days in a sealed container. But because it's so smooth, this mousse tastes best when it's still fresh.

- **Recipe 38: Coconut and Berry Chia Pudding**

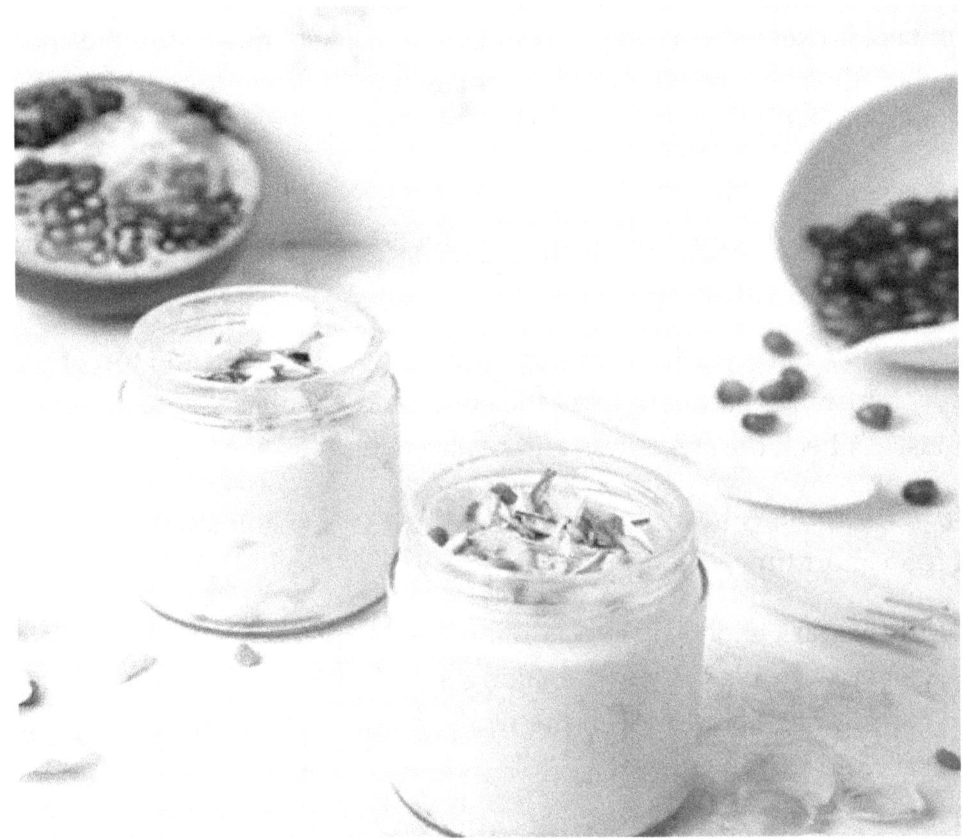

**Ingredients:**

*A Chia Pudding Recipe:*

- **Chia seeds, half a cup**

- **1.5 cups of full-fat coconut milk, either homemade or purchased, for added richness.**

- **Add two or three teaspoons of maple syrup, honey, or more if desired.**

- **Unsweetened vanilla extract, measuring one teaspoon. You may optionally add 1/4 cup of coconut shreds to add flavor and texture.**

**For the Berry Compote:**

- **Mixed Berries:** 1.5 cups of fresh or frozen berries (strawberries, blueberries, raspberries, etc.)

- **Honey or Maple Syrup:** 2 tablespoons (adjust to taste)

- **Lemon Juice:** 1 tablespoon (freshly squeezed)

**Optional Toppings:**

- **Fresh Berries:** For garnish

- **Sliced Almonds or Chopped Nuts:** For crunch (optional)

- **Mint Leaves:** For garnish (optional)

**Instructions:**

*For the Chia Pudding:*

1. *Combine Chia Seeds and Coconut Milk:* Combine the coconut milk and chia seeds in a mixing basin. Incorporate the chia seeds into the liquid well by vigorously churning them.

2. *Sweeten and Flavor:* Combine the coconut milk and chia seeds in a mixing basin. Incorporate the chia seeds into the liquid well by vigorously churning them.

3. *Set Aside to Thicken:* Place the bowl in the refrigerator for at least four hours, or ideally, all night.. Cover it with plastic wrap or a lid. During this time, the chia seeds will soak up the liquid, making the mixture thick and pudding-like.

4. *Add Shredded Coconut (Optional):* If you want, you can add the unsweetened shredded coconut right before serving or use it as a dessert.

**For the Berry Compote:**

1. *Prepare Berries:* Put the mixed berries, honey or maple syrup, and lemon juice in a different pot. Warm it up over medium-low heat.

2. ***Simmer and Mash:*** Let the mixture slowly cook for 10 to 15 minutes, or until the berries break down and the juices come out. You can mash the berries with a fork or a potato masher to make a thick sauce.

3. ***Cool:*** Leave the berry compote alone until it's cool enough to touch.

**Assembly:**

1. ***Layer Chia Pudding and Berry Compote:*** To serve, put a layer of the chia pudding into cups or bowls for each person. Add a big spoonful of the berry sauce on top of it.

2. ***Garnish:*** Garnish your coconut and berry chia pudding with fresh berries, sliced almonds, or chopped nuts for added texture and mint leaves for a pop of color and freshness.

3. ***Serve:*** Present your delightful creation as a healthy, satisfying breakfast or dessert. Enjoy the creamy coconut chia pudding layered with the sweet and tangy berry compote.

**Recipe Notes:**

- You can make this chia pudding your own by adding your favorite toppings, like granola, honey, or your best yogurt.

- You can change how sweet the chia pudding and berry sauce are by adding more or less honey or maple syrup.

- This dish is delicious, yet it's also packed with nutritious components. Chia seeds provide a lot of healthy fats and fiber, while berries are abundant in antioxidants and vitamins.

- Experiment with different berry combinations to suit your tastes or what's in season. Enjoy this Coconut and Berry Chia Pudding as a wholesome and satisfying treat.

- **Recipe 39: Baked Apples with Cinnamon**

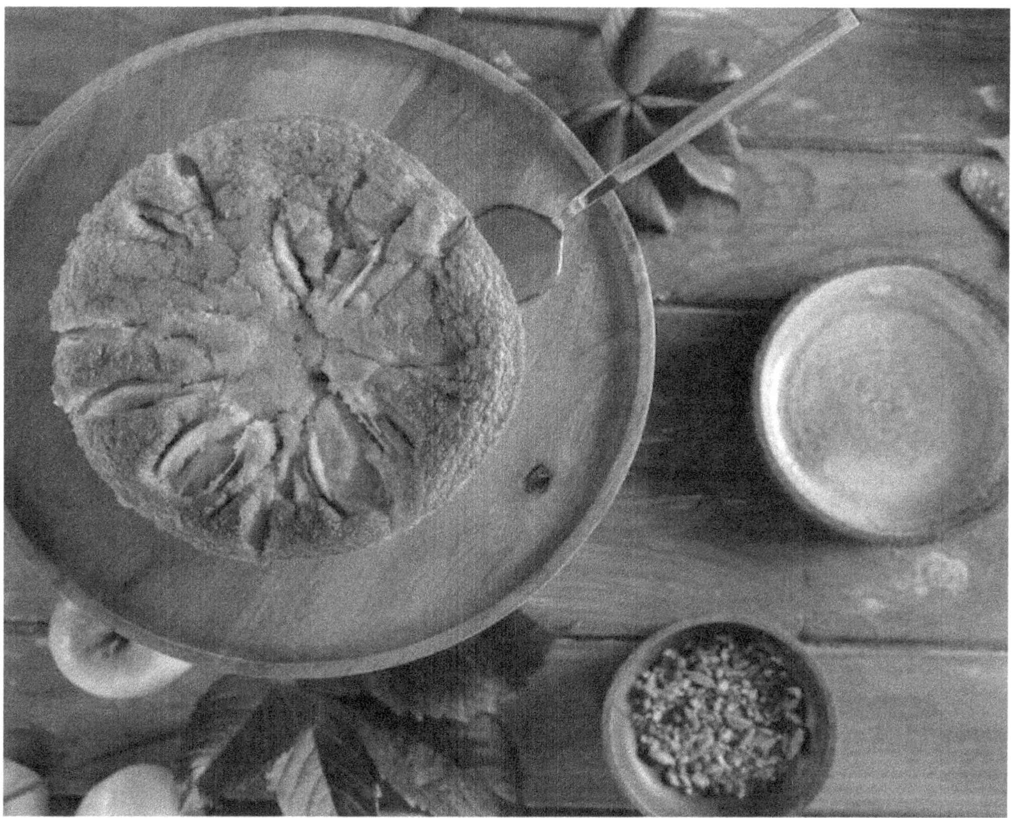

## Ingredients:

- **Apples:** 4 medium-sized apples (use a sweet variety like Honeycrisp or Gala)

- **Cinnamon:** 2 teaspoons

- **Brown Sugar:** 2 tablespoons (adjust to taste)

- **Butter:** 2 tablespoons (unsalted), divided into four equal portions

- **Raisins or Chopped Nuts:** 1/4 cup (optional, for added texture and flavor)

- **Lemon Juice:** 2 tablespoons (freshly squeezed to prevent browning)

- **Ice cream flavors: vanilla or whipped:** As a means of providing (not required)

## Instructions:

1. *Preheat the Oven:* Set oven temperature to 375°F, or 190°C.

2. *Prepare Apples:* Make sure to wash the apples well and then pat them dry. With a corer or a paring knife, remove the apple cores. Be careful not to slice through the apple core; you want to make a well in the middle.

3. *Lemon Juice:* Drizzle the freshly squeezed lemon juice over the apples. This helps prevent browning and adds a touch of brightness to the flavor.

4. *Fill the Apples:* Brown sugar and cinnamon should be combined in a small basin. Make four equal portions out of this mixture. Put a little bit into the apple's cavity. You may also garnish each apple with chopped nuts or dates.

5. *Dot with Butter:* On top of the cinnamon and sugar mix in each apple, put a small piece of butter (about 1/2 tbsp).

6. *Bake:* Put the apple stuffed with bacon in a baking dish. If the apples start to stick, you can put a little water or apple juice in the bottom of the dish. Take metal foil and put it over the dish.

7. After 30–40 minutes in the oven, the apples should be tender but not mushy. The precise duration could vary according to the kind and quantity of apples you use.

8. *Serve:* Take the apples out of the oven after they're done cooking and let them cool down a bit. Feel free to serve them warm on their own or with a scoop of vanilla ice cream or a dollop of whipped cream for an extra sweet treat.

9. *Enjoy:* As you slice into the juicy apple, breathe in the delightful aroma of cinnamon-baked apples. The warm, sugary, spicy filling complements the apple's sweetness.

**Recipe Notes:**

- THis method can be changed in many ways. You can try adding different fillings, like chopped nuts, dried fruits, or even honey or maple syrup, to make it sweeter.

- You can take off the paper for the last 10 to 15 minutes of baking to let the apples' tops brown a bit if you want a more browned and crispy top.

- Baked apples with cinnamon make for a simple and comforting dessert or snack, perfect for enjoying during the fall or any time of the year. They offer a warm and satisfying treat with minimal effort.

- Recipe 40: Turmeric Golden Milk Ice Cream

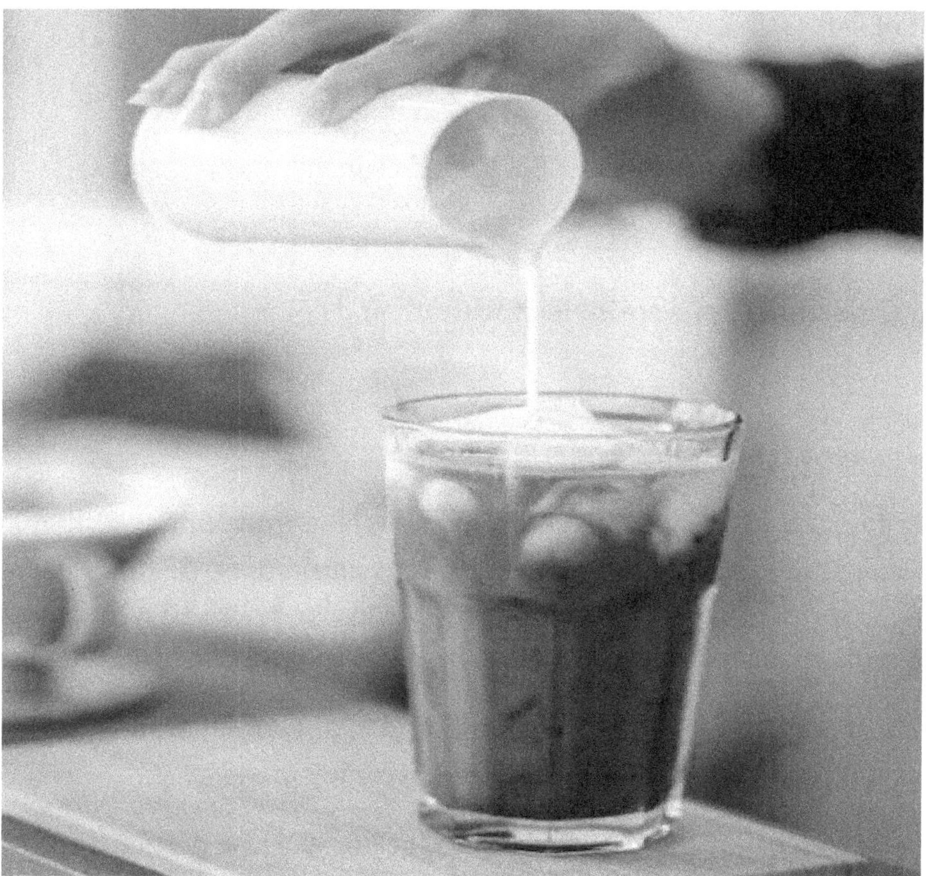

Ingredients:

*For the Turmeric Ice Cream Base:*

- Heavy cream, 2 cups

- One measuring cup of full-fat milk

- How much turmeric powder is required?

- A quarter teaspoon of cinnamon powder

- Half a teaspoon of ginger powder

- Ground cardamom, 1/4 teaspoon, will give it a delicious touch.

- To enhance turmeric absorption, add 1/4 teaspoon of ground black pepper.

- Half a cup of maple syrup or honey–or more, according to taste), should be used.

- **Vanilla essence, measuring one teaspoon**

- **A pinch of salt**

**For Garnish (Optional):**

- **Chopped Pistachios or Almonds:** For added crunch

- **Honey Drizzle:** For extra sweetness and presentation

- **Ground Cinnamon:** For a sprinkle of warmth and color

**Instructions:**

*Preparing the Turmeric Ice Cream Base:*

1. *Combine Ingredients:* In a bowl, combine the whole milk, honey or maple syrup, ground cinnamon, powdered ginger, ground cardamom (if desired), turmeric powder, a sprinkle of salt, and ground black pepper. Toss the ingredients together with a whisk. Before serving, whisk together all of the ingredients.

2. *Taste and Adjust:* You can taste the blend and change how sweet or spicy it is to your liking. If you need to, you can add more honey or spices.

3. *Chill the Mixture:* Put the bowl in the fridge for at least two to three hours, or until the mixture is completely cold. You can cover it with plastic wrap or a lid. Putting the ice cream in the fridge helps the flavors blend and makes sure it churns right.

**Churning the Ice Cream:**

1. *Prepare Your Ice Cream Maker:* Before churning, ensure your ice cream maker is cold according to the manufacturer's guidelines.

2. *Churn:* Make turmeric ice cream according to the manufacturer's instructions after adding the cold base to your maker. The typical cooking time is twenty to twenty-five minutes, and the finished product has a soft-serve texture.

**Finishing and Freezing:**

1. *Garnish (Optional):* While the mixture is still going, add chopped nuts or pistachios for an extra crunch.

2. *Transfer and Freeze:* Put the whipped ice cream in the freezer for at least four to six hours or until it reaches your desired consistency.

**Serving:**

1. *Scoop and Enjoy:* Put the turmeric golden milk ice cream into bowls or cones when it's hard. Add more chopped nuts if you want, then drizzle honey and ground cinnamon on top.

2. *Indulge:* Enjoy the unique flavors of this ice cream made from golden milk. The rich warmth of the turmeric and spices is mixed with the cool sweetness of the ice cream to make a tasty and refreshing treat.

**Recipe Notes:**

- Because I don't have an ice cream machine, put the chilled liquid in a container that can go in the freezer. For the first two to three hours, stir it every 30 minutes to break up the ice crystals and get the consistency you want.

- Turmeric is known for its bright color and stain-causing abilities. When working with turmeric, be careful and clean any surfaces or tools that get it on them right away.

- This turmeric golden milk ice cream is a unique and healthful dessert option, offering the anti-inflammatory benefits of turmeric alongside the creamy indulgence of ice cream. Enjoy its distinctive taste and cooling properties, especially during warm weather or as a soothing treat any time of the year

- **Recipe 41: Turmeric and Ginger Tea**

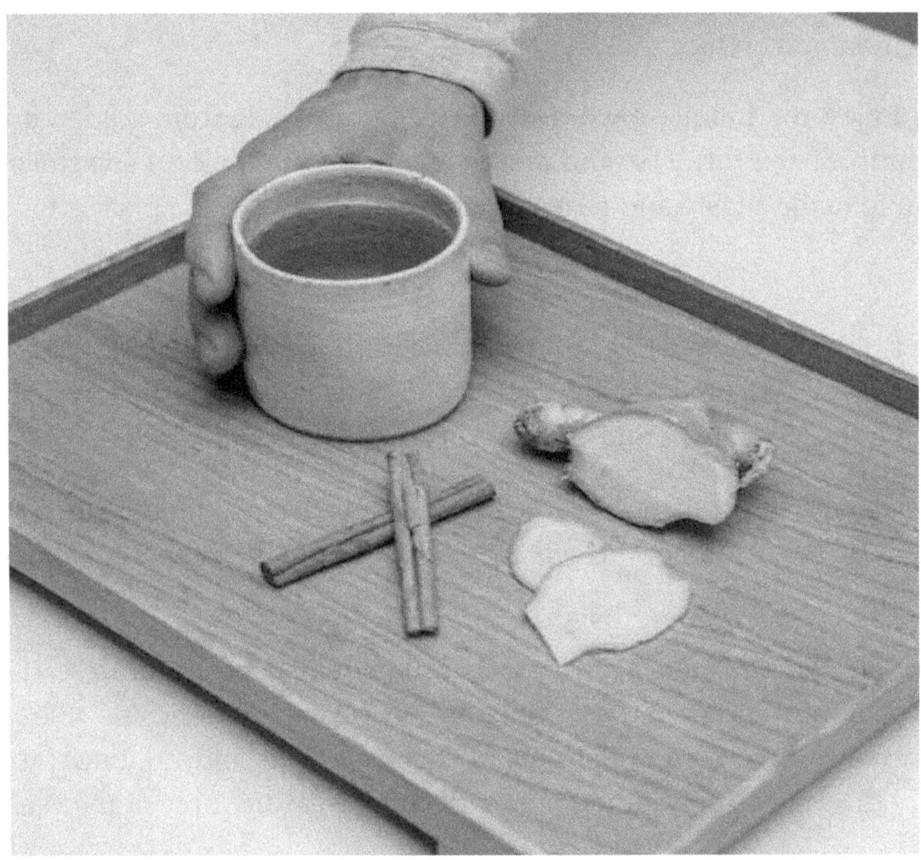

**Ingredients:**

- **Water:** 2 cups

- **Fresh Turmeric Root:** 1-inch piece, thinly sliced (or one teaspoon of ground turmeric)

- **Fresh Ginger Root:** 1-inch piece, thinly sliced (or one teaspoon of ground ginger)

- **Black Peppercorns:** 1/4 teaspoon (whole or crushed)

- **Honey:** 1-2 tablespoons (adjust to taste)

- **Lemon Juice:** 1-2 tablespoons (freshly squeezed, adjust to taste)

- ****Optional:** Cinnamon Stick, Cardamom Pods, or Cloves for added flavor variety

**Instructions:**

1. ***Prepare the Ingredients:*** Wash and peel the fresh turmeric and ginger roots if using. Slice them thinly to maximize the surface area for extraction of flavor and nutrients. If using ground turmeric and ginger, you can skip this step.

2. ***Boil Water:*** In a small pot, heat up 2 cups of water. For this step, you can also use an electric pot.

3. ***Add Turmeric and Ginger:*** Turn down the heat and add the ginger and turmeric slices (or ground turmeric and ginger if you want to use) once Once the water begins to boil, it will continue to boil fast.

4. ***Add Black Peppercorns:*** Put the black peppercorns into the pot. Curcumin, the main ingredient in turmeric, is better absorbed when black pepper is added.

5. ***Optional Spices:*** If you'd like to experiment with additional flavors, add a cinnamon stick, a few cardamom pods, or a couple of cloves to the mixture at this stage.

6. ***Simmer:*** For 10 to 15 minutes, let the turmeric and ginger tea slowly cook. Infusing the tastes into the water in this way.

7. ***Strain:*** As soon as the tea starts to bubble, take the pot off the heat and strain the tea to get rid of the lumps. If you use ground spices, Pour the tea into a tea infuser or strainer with a fine mesh.

8. ***Sweeten and Add Lemon:*** While the tea is still warm, sweeten it with honey, starting with 1-2 tablespoons, and add lemon juice, beginning with 1-2 tablespoons. Adjust the sweetness and acidity to your taste. Lemon juice provides a bright contrast to the earthy spices.

9. ***Stir and Serve:*** Stir the honey and lemon juice into the tea until fully dissolved. Your turmeric and ginger tea is now ready to be enjoyed.

10. ***Sip and Savor:*** Sip the warm and aromatic tea slowly, savoring its soothing and refreshing qualities. You can adjust the honey and lemon as needed during consumption.

**Recipe Notes:**

- Fresh turmeric and ginger provide the most vibrant flavors and beneficial compounds. However, ground versions work well when fresh ingredients are not available.

- Turmeric and ginger tea are good for you in many ways, like reducing inflammation and protecting cells from damage. It can help your immune system, ease stomach pain, and make you feel better by making a warm drink.

- Make ginger and turmeric tea according to your liking. Adjust the amount of honey, lemon, or spices to get your desired taste profile.

- Enjoy this tea as a comforting and healthful beverage at any time of the day, whether for its soothing qualities, as a pick-me-up or as part of your daily wellness routine.

- **Recipe 42: Smoothie with Berry Blast**

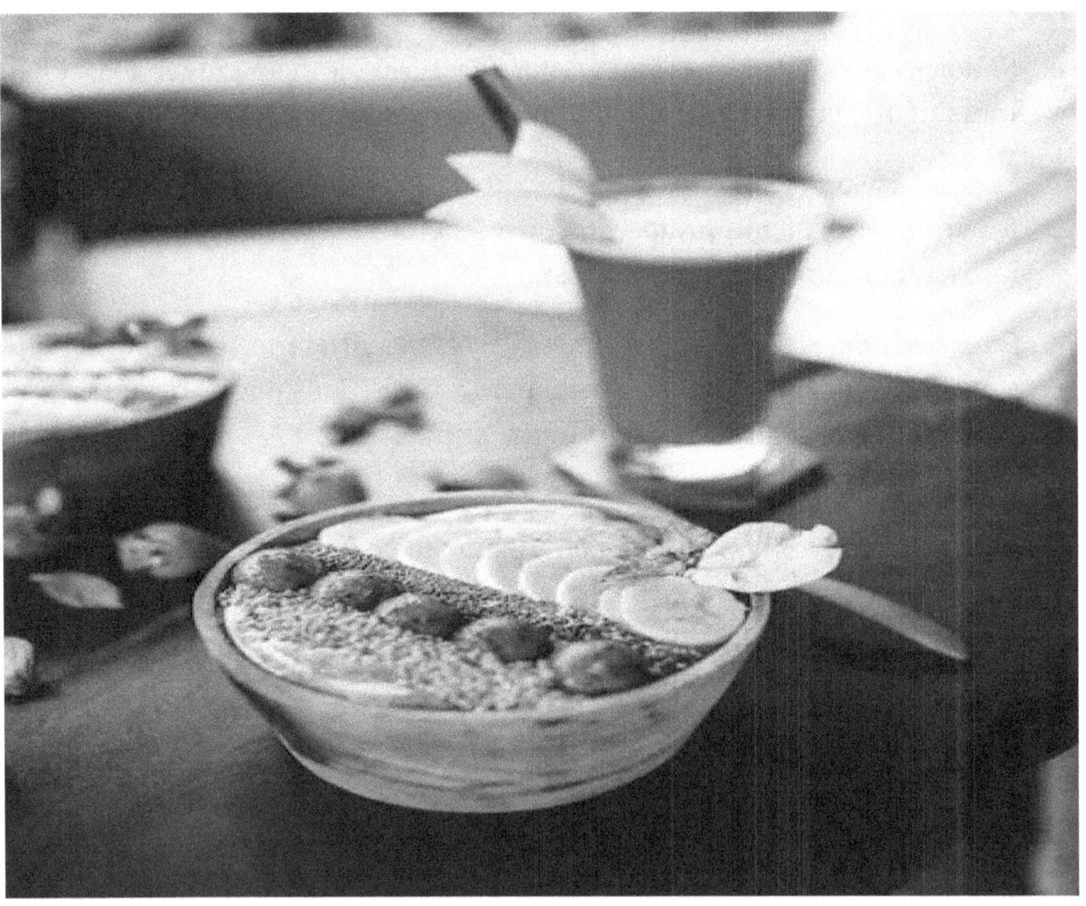

**Ingredients:**

- Mixed berries, one cup frozen

- Ripe banana: one ripe banana

- Either vanilla or plain Greek yogurt, measuring 1/2 cup, will do.

- To add calories, try adding 1 cup of either fresh or frozen kale or spinach.

- Add two or three teaspoons of maple syrup, honey, or more if desired.

- One cup of almond milk or more milk (thickness may be adjusted to taste).

- To increase the fiber and Omega-3s, add 1 tablespoon of chia seeds or flaxseeds.

- To make a thicker and colder smoothie, sprinkle in half a cup of ice cubes.

**Instructions:**

1. *Gather Ingredients:* Collect all the ingredients you'll need for your Berry Blast Smoothie.

2. *Prepare the Berries:* Use fresh berries, wash them in cold water, and take off any stems or leaves. Because the berries are frozen, you can use them right away.

3. *Combine Ingredients:* In a high-speed blender, add the frozen mixed berries, ripe banana, Greek yogurt, and fresh spinach or kale (if using). These ingredients form the core of your smoothie.

4. *Sweeten It Up:* Drizzle honey or maple syrup into the blender. The amount you use depends on your sweetness preference, so start with one tablespoon and adjust as needed.

5. *Add Chia or Flax Seeds:* Sprinkle chia seeds or flaxseeds on top to get even more fiber and Omega-3 oil. The drink is also thicker because of these seeds.

6. *Pour in Milk:* Pour in your choice of milk, whether it's almond milk, dairy milk, or any other plant-based milk you prefer. The amount of milk you use can be adjusted based on how thick or thin you want your smoothie.

7. *Optional Ice Cubes:* You can make it cooler and thicker by adding a few ice cubes to the blender.

8. ***Blend Until Smooth:*** Cover the blender and process the contents until a smooth consistency is achieved. Blend everything using the "smoothie" option for the smoothest results.

9. ***Taste and Adjust:*** Stop mixing and take a bite of the drink. Add more honey or maple syrup if you want it sweeter. Too thick? Add more milk. Too thin? Add more ice or frozen fruit.

10. ***Serve:*** Once the taste and texture are satisfied, pour your Berry Blast Smoothie into a glass or a to-go cup.

11. ***Garnish (Optional):*** Add some extra berries, a banana slice, or chia seeds to the top of your drink to make it look nicer.

12. ***Enjoy:*** Sip and enjoy your delicious and nutritious Berry Blast Smoothie as a refreshing breakfast, snack, or post-workout refuel.

**Recipe Notes:**

- You can make your Berry Blast Smoothie however you like. Adding a handful of spinach or kale won't change the taste much but will give you extra vitamins and minerals.

- Add more honey or maple syrup to make it as sweet as you like. The ripe banana and berries may be sweet enough for your taste buds on their own.

- You don't have to add chia seeds or flaxseeds, but you should because they are very good for you. They also make the drink thicker and give it a nice taste.

- This smoothie is delicious and packed with antioxidants, fiber, and vitamins from the mixed berries, making it a healthy and satisfying choice to kickstart your day or satisfy your cravings.

- **Recipe 43: Green Detox Juice**

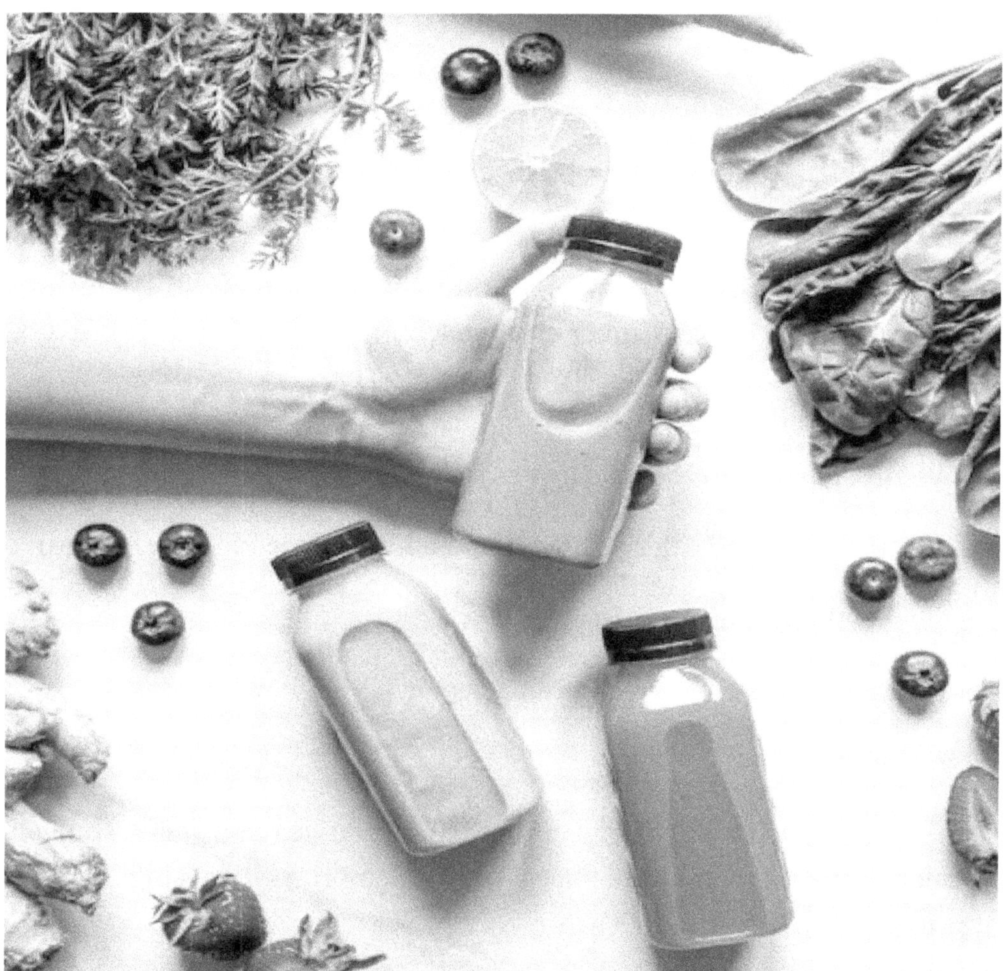

**Ingredients:**

- **Kale:** 2 large leaves (stems removed)

- **Spinach:** 1 cup (fresh)

- **Cucumber:** 1 medium (peeled if not organic)

- **Celery Stalks:** 2-3

- **Green Apple:** 1 (cored and sliced)

- **Lemon:** 1 (peeled and seeds removed)

- **Ginger:** 1-inch piece (peeled)

- **Fresh Mint Leaves:** A handful (optional, for added freshness)

* **Water:** 1/2 cup (for blending, adjust for desired consistency)

* **Ice Cubes:** For a colder juice (optional)

**Instructions:**

*1. Gather Ingredients:* Collect all the fresh and organic ingredients needed for your Green Detox Juice.

*2. Wash and Prep:* Wash all the vegetables and fruits thoroughly. If not using organic produce, consider peeling the cucumber and the lemon to reduce pesticide exposure.

**3. Prepare the Ingredients:**

* Remove the stems from the kale leaves.

* Slice the cucumber and celery stalks into smaller pieces for easier blending.

* Slice the green apple after coring it.

* Please get rid of the lemon's seeds and peel it.

* Peel the ginger.

*4. Blend:* In a high-speed blender, combine the kale leaves, fresh spinach, sliced cucumber, celery stalks, green apple slices, peeled lemon, peeled ginger, and optional fresh mint leaves.

*5. Add Water:* Put in half a cup of water. If you want the mixture to be lighter, you can add more water.

*6. Ice Cubes (Optional):* Put some ice cubes in the blender if you'd like your Green Detox Juice to be very cold.

*7. Blend Until Smooth:* Put the lid on the blender and mix the items together until you have a smooth, bright green juice. The time it takes may depend on how strong your blender is.

*8. Taste and Adjust:* Wait a minute and taste the juice. You can add a little honey or a small slice of green apple to make it tastier. Change the items to suit your taste.

*9. Strain (Optional):* If you'd rather have juice without the pulp, strain it into a glass or pitcher through a fine mesh strainer or a nut milk bag.

*10. Serve:* Pour your freshly made Green Detox Juice into a glass and serve immediately.

**11.** *Enjoy:* Sip and enjoy your nutrient-packed Green Detox Juice as a refreshing and healthful way to kickstart your day or as a midday pick-me-up.

**Recipe Notes:**

- For creaminess, you can customize this detox juice by adding other green vegetables like parsley, cilantro, or even a small slice of avocado.

- Fresh mint leaves are optional but can enhance the overall freshness and flavor of the juice.

- Adjust the sweetness to your liking. The green apple adds natural sweetness, but you can modify it with honey or another preferred sweetener.

- To get the most out of the health benefits of your Green Detox Juice, drink it soon after making it. It can be kept in the fridge for a few hours in a sealed container, but it tastes best when it's fresh.


- **Recipe 44: Anti-Inflammatory Golden Milk Latte**

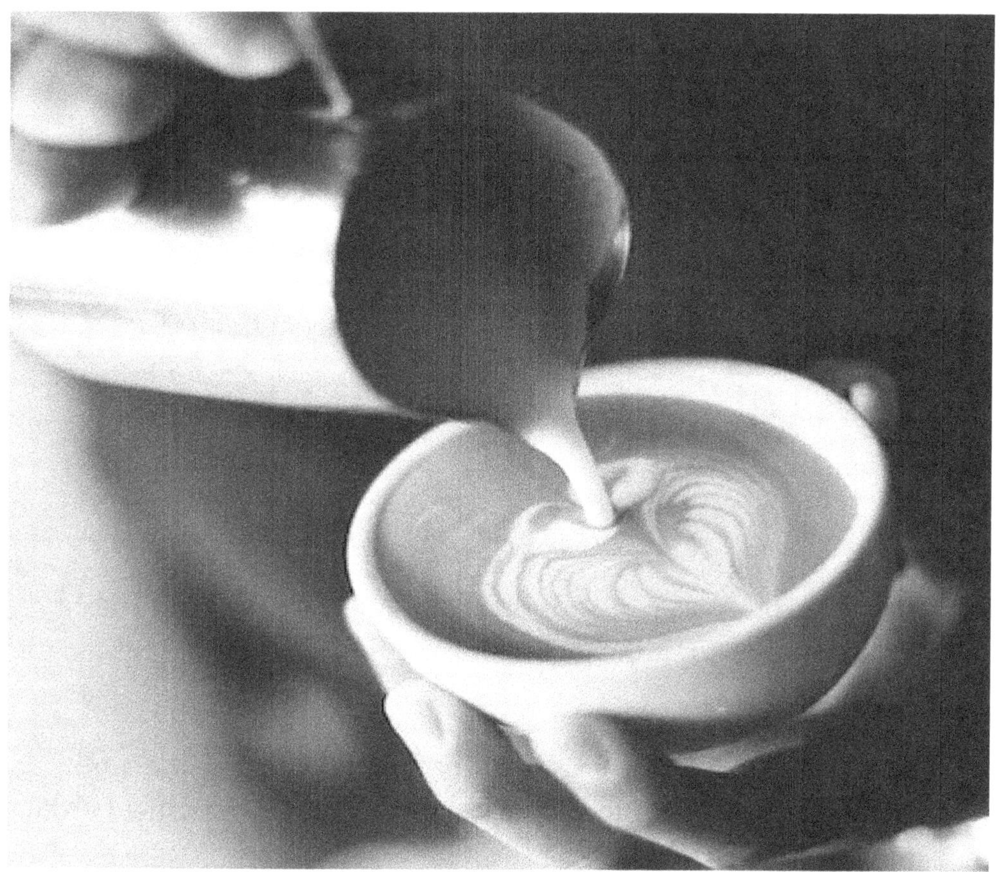

**Ingredients:**

*For the Golden Milk Base:*

- Turmeric, measuring half a teaspoon

- Half a teaspoon each of ground ginger and cinnamon

- Some ground black pepper (a pinch) helps the body absorb turmeric.

- Two to three tablespoons of honey or maple syrup, or as much as you like.

- Half a teaspoon of vanilla extract

- 1 teaspoon of coconut oil or ghee (for extra softness, if you want).

- One cup of almond milk or any other milk you like

**For Frothing and Topping:**

- **Espresso or Strong Coffee:** 1 shot (optional, for a latte-style drink)

- **Whipped Cream or Foam:** For topping (optional)

- **Ground Cinnamon or Nutmeg:** For garnish (optional)

**Instructions:**

*1. Gather Ingredients:* Collect all the ingredients needed for your Anti-Inflammatory Golden Milk Latte.

*2. Prepare the Golden Milk Base:*

- Put some ground black pepper, honey or maple syrup, vanilla extract, ground cinnamon, ground ginger, and turmeric powder in a small pot. If you want to use ghee or coconut oil, do so now.

- Use any milk you like to add to the bowl.

*3. Heat and Stir:* Put the saucepan over medium-low heat and constantly swirl the ingredients. Heat it, but avoid boiling it. The milk could curl if heated for too long, so be cautious.

*4. Frothing (Optional):* If your latte has a frothy texture, you can use a milk frother to froth the golden milk mixture. Alternatively, you can use a handheld frother or an immersion blender.

**5. *Espresso (Optional):*** If you prefer a latte-style drink, brew a shot of espresso or prepare a strong cup of coffee.

**6. *Combine and Serve:***

- Pour the hot espresso or coffee into a latte glass.

- Carefully pour the frothy golden milk mixture over the coffee, holding back the foam with a spoon if necessary.

**7. *Top with Foam or Whipped Cream (Optional):*** For a fancy touch, you can add whipped cream or foam on top of your latte if you'd like.

**8. *Garnish (Optional):*** Sprinkle a pinch of ground cinnamon or nutmeg on top for extra flavor and presentation.

**9. *Serve:*** Your Anti-Inflammatory Golden Milk Latte is ready to enjoy.

**10. *Sip and Savor:*** Sip your comforting and healthful latte slowly, savoring the golden milk base's warm, soothing flavors and potential anti-inflammatory benefits.

**Recipe Notes:**

- Customize your Golden Milk Latte by adjusting the sweetness to your liking. You can add more honey or maple syrup for a sweeter taste.

- Coconut oil or ghee adds creaminess to the latte but is optional. You can omit it if you prefer a lighter drink.

- If you don't have espresso or coffee, you can drink the golden milk base whenever you want, like before bed or first thing in the morning.

- Incorporating the anti-inflammatory qualities of turmeric, cinnamon, and ginger into your daily routine makes you more cozy with this latte.

- Experiment with different milk alternatives, such as almond, coconut, or oat milk, to find your favorite flavor combination.

- **Recipe 45: Cucumber and Mint Infused Water**

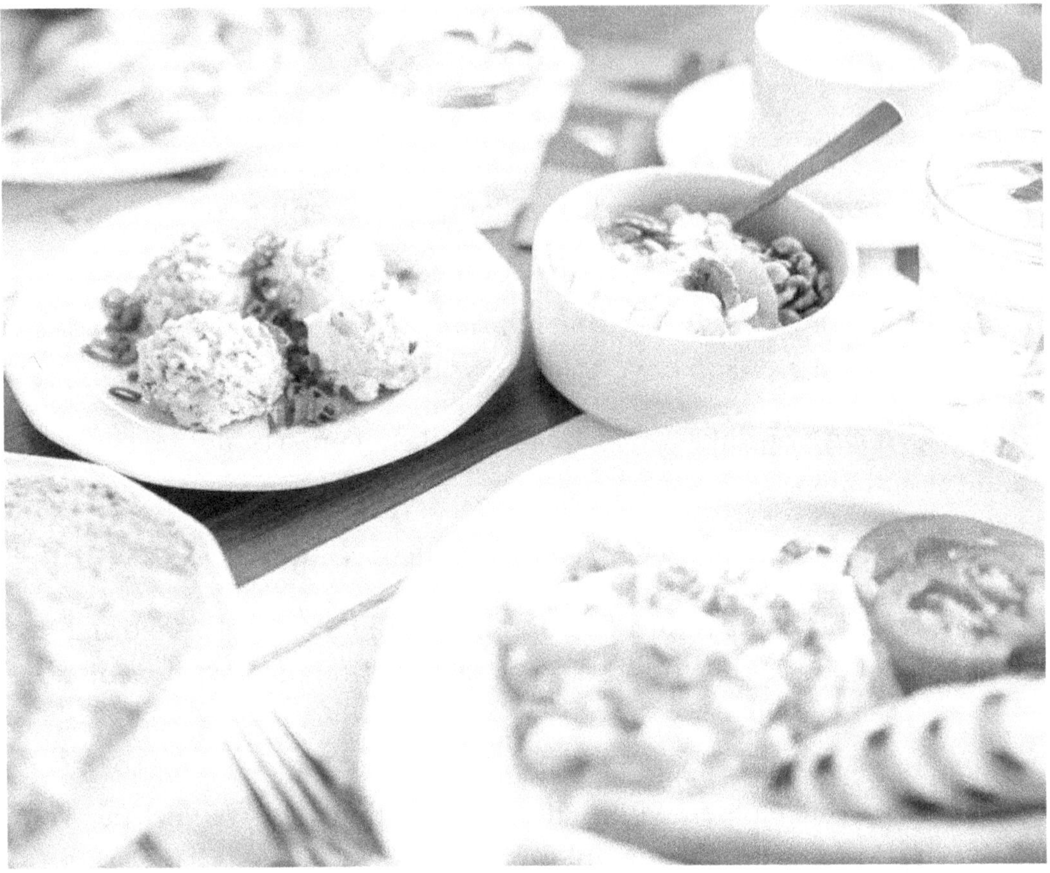

**Ingredients:**

- **Cucumber:** 1 medium cucumber, preferably organic

- **Fresh Mint Leaves:** A small handful, about 10-12 leaves

- **Water:** 8 cups (2 liters), filtered for the best taste

- **Ice Cubes**: Optional for a colder infusion

**Instructions:**

*1. Wash and Prepare Ingredients:*

- Wash the cucumber thoroughly to remove any pesticides or dirt, especially if it's not organic.

- Slice the cucumber into thin rounds or ribbons. You can use a knife or a mandoline slicer for this. Leave the skin on, as it adds flavor and nutrients.

*2. Tear Mint Leaves:*

- Gently tear the fresh mint leaves with your hands. This releases the natural oils and flavors, enhancing the infusion.

*3. Combine Ingredients:*

- Put the cut cucumber slices and torn mint leaves in a big bowl or glass jar.

*4. Add Water:*

- Pour 8 cups (2 liters) of filtered Water over the cucumber and mint in the pitcher.

*5. Optional: Add Ice Cubes:*

- If you want your infused Water to be extra refreshing, add ice cubes to the pitcher or directly to your glass when serving.

*6. Infuse:*

- Gently mix the ingredients to distribute the flavors. Chill the water with the mint and cucumber for at least an hour before serving. The flavor will really come through after a few hours or perhaps overnight in the fridge.

*7. Serve:*

- Pour the infused Water into glasses or a water bottle when ready to enjoy it.

*8. Garnish (Optional):*

- For a visually appealing presentation, add a few cucumber slices and mint leaves to each glass.

*9. Sip and Enjoy:*

- Sip your refreshing cucumber and mint-infused Water throughout the day. It's a delightful and hydrating way to stay cool and enjoy a subtle infusion of flavors.

**Recipe Notes:**

- Customize the intensity of the flavors by adjusting the cucumber and mint quantities to your taste preferences. Some people prefer a stronger infusion, while others like it more subtle.

- This infused Water is perfect for staying hydrated and especially refreshing on hot days or after a workout.

- Feel free to reuse the cucumber and mint for a second batch of infused Water. Add more water to the pitcher and enjoy another round of refreshing hydration.

- Adding a touch of minty freshness to water while maintaining a crisp, clean flavor, cucumber and mint make a traditional infusion. This is a fantastic option if you're looking for a way to spice up your water intake without adding sugar.

- This cucumber and mint-infused Water is not only delicious but also healthy. Cucumber provides hydration and vitamins, while mint adds a burst of flavor without any added calories or sugar.

**Conclusion**

Through the use of food, this book provides a holistic approach to well-being. We have examined the transformational power of an anti-inflammatory diet throughout this book, leading you on a culinary adventure that not only reduces inflammation but also entices the senses.

In addition to numerous comforts, the contemporary world has brought about foods and habits that often encourage chronic inflammation. Numerous health problems, including arthritis, heart disease, digestive problems, and autoimmune diseases, are caused by this persistent inflammation. The ideas presented in this cookbook's recipes and advice are evidence that we can manage our health by making wise food choices.

By focusing on anti-inflammatory foods, you are not only controlling inflammation, but also living a lifestyle that boosts energy, resiliency, and lifespan. You now know that foods like fatty fish, bright berries, fresh greens, and spices like turmeric can help you take better care of your health. You now know that getting healthy doesn't mean giving up tasty foods or missing out on the pleasure of tasty meals.

We've delved deeply into the foods that may improve your well-being throughout this book. We've shown how to create delectable, health-improving meals, demonstrating that pursuing vitality can be a pleasurable journey. You've started along the road to culinary mastery, where the items you choose will have a big impact on your general well-being and pleasure.

Keep in mind that leading an anti-inflammatory lifestyle is about release, not constraint. It's about embracing the limitless energy, the enthusiasm for life, and the health you deserve and releasing yourself from the chains of chronic inflammation. You have the chance to feed your body, reduce inflammation, and enjoy the pleasure of fine cuisine with each meal you create with the recipes in this cookbook.

Use this book as a starting point for your culinary journey into the realm of anti-inflammatory cuisine. Play around with the recipes, discover new tastes, and personalize them. Share the culinary discoveries you make with the people you care about since this fosters a feeling of satisfaction and community.

It's always possible to make investments in your health, which is your most valuable possession. You now have the necessary tools, thanks to this cookbook, to gradually improve your health while enjoying tasty meals. But keep in mind that living an anti-inflammatory lifestyle goes beyond your dinner. For a comprehensive approach to well-being, include regular physical exercise, control stress, and promote restful sleep.

The ultimate objective is to develop a bright, balanced, and sustainable existence in addition to reducing inflammation. So, when you enjoy your final mouthful of a delicious anti-inflammatory dinner, take comfort in the fact that you've made considerable progress toward being a healthier, happier version of yourself.

Cheers to your route to a life free of chronic inflammation, well-being, and the innumerable delectable meals that lie ahead of you. May every mouthful bring you happiness and contentment, and may you enjoy the many health advantages that lie ahead.